*"I tried every diet there was! Nothing worked until phen-Prozac. I was totally disabled until I lost 92 pounds. I am now walking five miles a day and will start my own business shortly. Thanks so much for telling me about phen-Prozac."*

**Cynthia Frye, 92 pounds lost**

*"From day one, I was afraid to prescribe fenfluramine to my overweight patients because of the risks described in the* Physicians' Desk Reference. *With the recent news linking heart and lung disease to phen-fen, Dr. Anchors's alternative looks like the good news millions of overweight people have been waiting for!"*

**Helen Pensanti, M.D., host of the TV show *Doctor to Doctor***

*"I weighed 283 pounds two years ago when Dr. Anchors prescribed phentermine . . . and Prozac to help control my appetite. A sensible, nutritious diet combined with regular exercise, long walks, and [workout] videos have resulted in a gradual weight loss of over 100 pounds. Now I can enjoy wearing pretty clothes and feel good about myself."*

**Deb White, 154 pounds lost**

*"It has been a godsend. I am not eating just to eat. I am eating when I am hungry and my body does the rest."*

**Todd Bardwell, 22 pounds lost so far**

*"After losing 46 pounds by following Dr. Anchors's plan, my diabetes disappeared."*

**David Sampson, 46 pounds lost**

*"I used phen-Prozac to lose 126 pounds in a year and reached my ideal body weight. None of the diets ever worked for me before. I have kept the weight off for a year, exercising frequently. I am one of the lucky patients who does not need to keep taking the medicines."*

**Glenn Darby, 126 pounds lost**

*"Since 1995 I have treated patients with the combination [detailed in this book] of Zoloft and phentermine, reducing the total weight of my practice by more than 10,000 pounds. I am extremely excited about the results and feel this combination of medications is much safer and more effective than phen-fen!"*

**Ronald J. Hamm, M.D.**

*"I started taking phentermine and Prozac on Friday, April 11, 1997. On Saturday, I organized my closet, arranging my size 12 to 18 clothing, and, as I recall, that span in size started in 1994. I was excited and energetic and looked forward to any weight loss.*

*"This morning I put on a size 14 suit—a little tight but still a 14. This weekend the fat clothes will be put away and I plan to start a light workout."*

**Kathryn Helton, 32 pounds lost so far**

*"I was always hungry. I thought about food constantly, but I knew my health was in danger. I've been taking phen-Prozac for a year. I have more energy and a much lighter appetite."*

**Alan Driggs, 73 pounds lost**

# Safer Than Phen-Fen!

**Michael Anchors, M.D., Ph.D.**
*Member of the American Society of Bariatric Physicians*

Prima Publishing

**DISCLAIMER**

The reading of this book does not establish a doctor-patient relationship between the reader and Dr. Anchors. The reason there is a chapter in this book for physicians is precisely because Dr. Anchors wants overweight readers to consult their personal physicians for advice and medication.

The production of this work was not underwritten in any way by the pharmaceutical companies whose products are mentioned.

The information provided in this book is not intended to be a substitute for professional or medical advice. Publisher disclaims any warranty or representation, express or implied, regarding the information contained herein. The author and publisher specifically disclaim any liability, loss, or risk, personal or otherwise, that is incurred as a result, directly or indirectly, of the use and application of any of the contents of this book.

**Library of Congress Cataloging-in-Publication Data**

Anchors, Michael.

Safer than phen-fen! / Michael Anchors.

p. cm.

Includes bibliographical references and index.

ISBN 0-7615-1149-0

1. Phentermine. 2. Fluoxetine. 3. Obesity—Chemotherapy. 4. Fenfluramine—Side effects. 5. Dexfenfluramine—Side effects. 6. Serotonin reuptake inhibitors. 7. Pulmonary hypertension. I. Title.

RC628.A49 1997

616.3'98061—dc21 97-15285

CIP

97 98 99 00 01 HH 10 9 8 7 6 5 4 3 2 1

Printed in the United States of America

**How to Order**

Single copies may be ordered from Prima Publishing, P.O. Box 1260BK, Rocklin, CA 95677; telephone (916) 632-4400. Quantity discounts are also available. On your letterhead, include information concerning the intended use of the books and the number of books you wish to purchase.

**Visit us online at www.primapublishing.com**

*This book is dedicated to my patients, from whom I have learned so much about what is really important.*

# Contents

# An Important Medical Note to Readers

On pages 57 and 58 of this book I predicted that in addition to causing primary pulmonary hypertension (PPH), fenfluramine (also known as Pondimin or Redux) would also be found to cause heart valve disease and explained the reasons for my prediction. On July 8, 1997, two weeks before this book went to press, the news media broke the story that Dr. Heidi Connolly and colleagues at the Mayo Clinic had found twenty-four patients who had taken the older form of the phen-fen combination and developed serious heart valve disease, exactly as I had predicted. The new form of phen-fen described in this book, in which fenfluramine is replaced by Prozac, Zoloft, or Luvox, does not cause heart valve disease, nor does it cause PPH. The actual article in the *New England Journal of Medicine* in which Dr. Connolly's findings are described will not appear until August 1997, after this book is on its way to bookstores.

The particular heart valve involved is the mitral valve, the large flap-valve between the upper part of the heart and the lower part, on the left side. Blood returning from the lungs passes through this valve into the lower part of the heart before being pumped back to the body. If this valve fails, the forward flow of blood is interrupted. Unless the damaged valve is replaced by a difficult surgery, the patient may be so impaired that she cannot exercise or may even die.

If you have been taking fenfluramine in either of its forms, Pondimin or Redux, you might ask your doctor to check if you have a heart murmur. A test called an echocardiogram may need to be done to ascertain if you have heart valve disease. If you already have symptoms of shortness of breath, irregular heart beat, or chest pain, you should certainly consult your doctor.

Millions of patients have taken fenfluramine and only twenty-four cases of heart valve disease have been reported so far. Hopefully, it will turn out to be a rare problem, but you should take no chances.

And you should read this book.

Michael Anchors, M.D., Ph.D.

# Foreword

It's Oscar night. The parade of limousines unloading beautiful ultra-groomed celebrities has begun. Look! There's Sharon Stone! Wait, it's Mel Gibson, Tom Cruise, and wow, there's . . . Each star is more picture-perfect than the last. The whiter-than-bleach teeth, the high-gloss hairdos, the perfect gowns with those ribbons. What? Ribbons? Certainly you have noticed these tiny, colored nylon symbols of Hollywood's concern and care adorning your favorite star. Think of them as modern-day equivalents to the campaign ribbons embellishing the uniforms of Russian generals of the past world war. The red ribbon represents the battle against AIDS, which claims about 100 lives per day in the United States. The pink ribbon stands for breast cancer, to which 200 women fall victim every day.

Nevertheless, there is one ribbon missing. Where is the ribbon for obesity, which can result in ill health or death from diabetes, heart disease, arthritis, stroke, gallstones, or cancer? That Hollywood pays obesity so little attention comes as no surprise, for Tinseltown is the land of the thin. We adore the stars for their shapes, but the shape of things to come for sixty thousand obese Americans is not glamorous. They spend every day battling extra weight and hoping to avoid becoming the next victim of high blood pressure, diabetes, stroke, or heart attack. For increasing numbers of overweight people, the standard fare of dieting and health club memberships is not working. High-carbohydrate, low-fat, high-protein diets—it makes no difference. We get heavier as a nation with each passing day. A new pathway to weight loss and better health is sorely needed—one that can be followed by all overweight Americans. This is the path you have just begun by reading *Safer Than Phen-Fen.*

This book would not be possible without the explosion in understanding the causes of obesity that has occurred in the past few years. Being overweight, it turns out, has little to do with laziness or lack of willpower. Obesity is not a result of habits. Instead, obesity is a genetic, biochemical disorder of the brain. Through no fault of their own, overweight people have inherited different levels of hormones and receptors in their brains, causing them to be persistently hungry. Blaming obese people because they can't lose weight is about as sensible as blaming people in wheelchairs because they can't walk.

With this new understanding comes new ability to treat obesity. Doctors have been prescribing the weight-loss drugs Redux and phen-fen (a combination of phentermine and fenfluramine) in increasing numbers with varying rates of success. These medications control the appetite by raising levels of the appropriate hormones in the brain, and weight loss occurs as a result of diminished caloric intake. But studies have shown that phen-fen and Redux are not consistently effective, and they carry a risk of primary pulmonary hypertension (PPH), a serious lung disorder. You may have heard about PPH in the news.

Dr. Michael Anchors has taken the use of these types of medications to the next level. Drawing on his background as both an M.D. and a Ph.D. in biochemistry, Dr. Anchors noted the similarity between fenfluramine and the SSRI (Selective

Serotonin Reuptake Inhibitors) class of medicines, which includes Prozac, Luvox, and Zoloft. With his vision and concern for safety, he substituted low doses of Prozac for fenfluramine in the phen-fen combination. The new combination is effective and results in fewer side effects than phen-fen or Redux, and it carries no risk of PPH.

Hundreds of obese people have charted courses of success by following Dr. Anchors's weight-loss regimen along with modest lifestyle changes. His original patients were pioneers, and by following the weight-loss plan outlined in this book, you can join them. You can reach a healthy weight without suffering the side effects and problems of other weight-loss medications.

Dr. Anchors's lively style reflects a caring "old-fashioned" doctor who shares the same wishes as his readers: he wants everyone who is overweight to lose weight the smart and healthy way.

Enjoy the book, grasp the pioneer spirit, and, above all, don't be afraid of change. Perhaps we will never need that third ribbon after all . . .

Sheldon Levine, M.D.

# Acknowledgments

First, I want to thank my patients; through them I first learned of the phen-fen program, and it was their successful weight loss that proved the benefits of phen-Prozac to me. I must also acknowledge Janice Lester, the librarian at Shady Grove Adventist Hospital, for the many hours she spent poring through her computer database of scientific literature for me. Dr. Michael Weintraub was very kind in accepting the original invitation to lecture to physicians at our hospital; we all owe him a debt of gratitude. Dr. Richard Rothman, clinical director of the Be-Lite Medical Centers, shared with me his experience with three thousand patients on combination appetite-suppressant therapy.

Dr. Mark Eig, a physician in Silver Spring, Maryland, furnished me with several interesting insights into phen-fen. Dr. Gabe Mirkin, radio personality and author, encouraged me and kept me from feeling lonely in my opinions. Dr. Sheldon Levine, author of *The Redux Revolution*, and my friend, Dr. Uzi Ben-Ami, psychologist, reassured me that this book was worth the effort.

My family was enormously patient. My wife, Laurel, and my daughters never complained while I spent so much time at the computer. I wanted this book to be successful so that my oldest daughter, a journalism major in college, could see that America listens to writers.

My greatest thanks go to Prima Publishing for being willing to listen to new ideas with an open mind.

# Terms to Know

This book contains a wealth of information about weight-loss therapies that involve a variety of medications. Since many of these terms may be new to you, the following list gives you a quick introduction to the medications and related words you will be reading about.

**Appestat** (ap'-eh-stat). The appetite center in the brain that controls when you feel hungry and when you feel full.

**Fenfluramine** (fen-flur'-a-meen). The second most commonly used appetite-supressant medication in the United States and the most commonly used in French-speaking countries. Available since about 1974.

**Phen-fen.** Combined oral therapy for obesity using phentermine and fenfluramine, first promoted by Dr. Weintraub in 1992.

**Phen-Prozac.** An improved combination using Prozac instead of fenfluramine. First described publicly in this book.

**Phentermine** (fen'-ter-meen). The most commonly used appetite suppressant medication in the United States and Germany since 1970. Brand names in the United States are Adipex, Ionamin, and Fastin.

**Pondimin** (pond'-i-min). The first available brand of fenfluramin. Originally produced by the A. H. Robins company, it has since been taken over by the Wyeth-Ayerst company.

**PPH** (primary pulmonary hypertension). A rare, often fatal lung disorder in which the blood vessels in the lungs are destroyed. Fenfluramine, but not the SSRI class of medicines, increases the chance of getting PPH. Hence, phen-Prozac is safer than phen-fen.

**Redux** (ree'-dux). A new, more purified form of fenfluramine, available since April 1996. Product of Wyeth-Ayerst.

**SSRI.** The class of medicines to which **Prozac** belongs. Prozac is the most prominent member of the class. SSRI stands for Selective Serotonin Reuptake Inhibitor.

**Zoloft, Luvox, and trazodone.** Other SSRI medicines that work with phentermine to control obesity.

CHAPTER ONE

# Facing Up to Obesity

Knowledge is power, especially when it comes to your health. The more you know about a medical treatment, the better able you are to make informed decisions and discuss them with your doctor. This book will help you understand the health risks of obesity, the research behind weight-loss drugs and how they work, and why the combination of the medicines phentermine and Prozac is safe and effective for weight loss. What you learn in these pages may be the first step on the road to a healthier, thinner life.

## Breakthrough Discoveries

As a doctor, I am continually learning as new breakthroughs in medicine are discovered. Several years ago, before I knew much about medications for weight-loss, I faced obese patients in my office and simply "counseled" them on diet and exercise, saying only a few words and writing in the chart "low-fat diet discussed, patient told to exercise." I never pursued the matter beyond those steps.

And, of course, it never worked. The patients returned to my office over and over, as heavy as ever, and I still wrote the same useless words in the chart. Why didn't I pause to wonder why so many intelligent, motivated people could not lose weight and keep it off? Did they all, indeed, have a fault of character? Would any of them have chosen to be so obese if they could control it?

Fortunately, more clever people than myself were doing research at the time. They discovered what we all might have suspected all along: Obese people are not just thin people who overeat. They are not lazy or undisciplined. Through no fault of their own, their brains are biochemically different. Obese people are persistently hungry, and therein lies their problem—they have to eat more than they need in order to feel full (see Chapter 2 for more details). It is a chemical problem, and it has a chemical answer. The medicines to fix the problem have been around for thirty years, but no one recognized how they could be used for weight-loss until relatively recently. It remains now to find the best and safest way to use the medicines. That is what this book is about, the best way to use these weight-reducing medications. If you have ever struggled with obesity, or you love someone who has, this book is for you.

You are probably aware that obesity is a growing health problem in the United States. You may also have heard that some relatively new drug therapies—notably phen-fen and Redux—have revolutionized the field of weight-loss treatment. Phen-fen is the combination of phentermine and fenfluramine, two well-known weight-loss drugs that have been available individually for thirty years. Redux is a more-purified form of fenfluramine. But these medications have been known to have unpleasant and potentially fatal side effects. Both Redux and the fenfluramine component of phen-fen can cause heart valve disease and a fatal lung disorder called PPH (primary pulmonary hypertension; see Chapter 4).[1] These side effects do not occur frequently, but they are serious problems nevertheless. Patients with PPH have high blood pressure in their lungs, leading to congestive heart failure, asphyxia, and death. Most victims of PPH are young women.

Fortunately, there is a solution. The fenfluramine in the phen-fen combination can be replaced with Prozac or a similar medicine. Phen-Prozac is as effective as phen-fen in producing weight loss, and it confers no risk of PPH or heart valve disease. I have personally treated more than five hundred patients with this combination. Only seven patients failed to lose weight and eight had to discontinue the program because of side effects. There have been no serious side effects. The minor side effects that have occurred are listed in the final chapter, along with measures found to eliminate them.

The dose of Prozac used with phentermine in phen-Prozac is lower than the dose typically used to treat depression. Side effects from Prozac seldom occur; the side effects that do occur are a result of phentermine and they are manageable. We'll discuss phen-Prozac in more detail in Chapters 5 and 6.

My patients on phen-Prozac have lost an average of six pounds per month for as long as they take the therapy. Some have lost more than one hundred pounds! I have treated some overweight patients for as long as two years, and I will continue to treat them as long as necessary to keep the weight off. High body weight is as life-threatening as high blood pressure or high blood sugar. Obesity has a biochemical basis, and the answer to treating obesity is mainly chemical. What a pleasant surprise for the many overweight people who have been tortured by derision and guilt. The twenty-first century is dawning for them with good news.

*Obesity has a biochemical basis, and the answer to treating obesity is mainly chemical.*

I published an article for the scientific community at about the same time as this book went to press.[2] I felt it was important to publish this information in the lay press as well, to persuade physicians and patients to consider phen-Prozac instead of phen-fen and Redux, before any more people are put at risk for PPH and heart valve disease.

## What's So Bad About Being Overweight?

Most of us have become so used to seeing overweight people that we are immune to it. We overlook the fact that obesity is a serious health problem. Think about it—there is a reason why Stan Laurel outlived Oliver Hardy, why actor John Candy dropped dead on a movie set, why umpire John McSherry collapsed on the baseball field. The world is not a mean and random place; most people don't die for no reason. Those deaths were preventable.

When Dr. Michael Weintraub, the inventor of phen-fen, gave a talk at my local hospital, he began by observing that none of the obese patients in the original Framingham study is still alive. The Framingham study was the study, begun in the 1960s, of the adult inhabitants of Framingham, Massachusetts, from which most of our knowledge about the effects of smoking, high blood pressure, high cholesterol, and obesity is derived. By 1995, none of the obese participants in the study was alive!

Dr. Weintraub's observation meshed with my own experiences with elderly people in nursing homes; very few are obese. Why? You might think it is because their appetites are lower, or their teeth are worse, or they are fed a more balanced diet, but the fact is, few obese patients live long enough to enter a nursing home. For the same reason, there are fewer people with high blood pressure and fewer smokers in nursing homes than in the general population.

For an arresting picture of how obesity increases the risk of developing serious health conditions, see Figure 1.1.

Obesity increases the chance of heart attack and stroke, and many obese people have high cholesterol and high blood pressure as well. Any controversy surrounding the notion that obesity is unhealthy revolves around the question of whether obese people are unhealthy because of the obesity per se, or because of the high cholesterol, high blood pressure, diabetes,

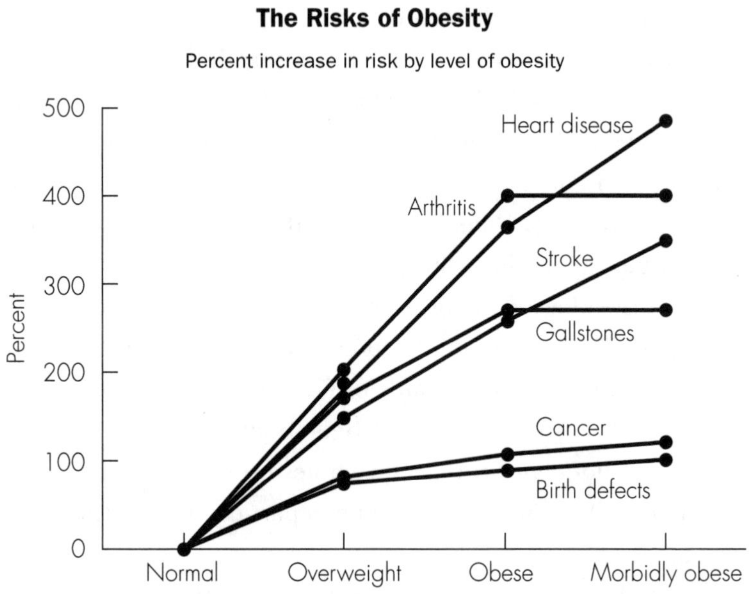


FIGURE 1.1

gout, and other conditions that often attend obesity.[3] It is pointless to try to resolve such a question; it's like arguing over how many angels can fit on the head of a pin. There are no healthy obese people. Period.

Obese individuals have an increased risk of cancer, particularly of the colon and breast. In one study, women who are morbidly obese (see page 10 for definition) had four times the risk of death from coronary artery disease and twice the risk of death from cancer compared to normal weight women.[4] As shown in Figure 1.2, the chance of developing diabetes mellitus increases 5000 percent in morbidly obese people. (See Chapter 10 for further discussion of obesity-related health problems.)

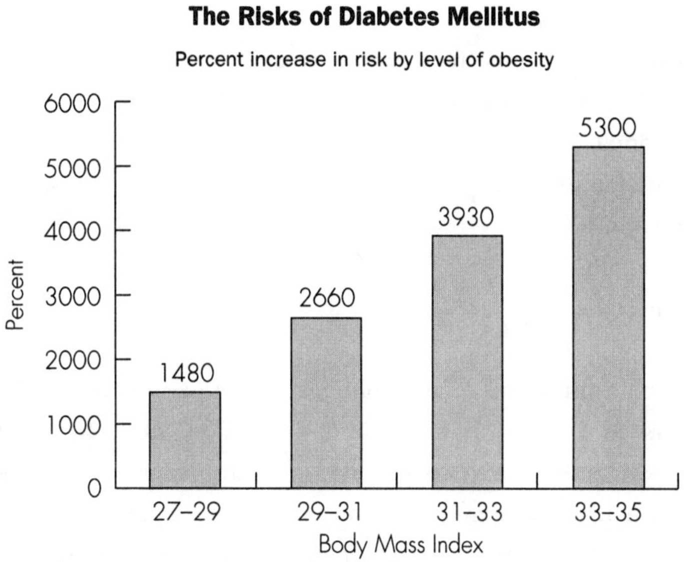


FIGURE 1.2

**Conditions Made Worse by Obesity**

asthma
blood clots in legs
breast growth in men
cancer
complications during pregnancy
congestive heart failure
dark pigment on legs
depression
diabetes mellitus
diverticulosis
fatty liver
gout
heart disease

heavy, irregular menstrual periods
high blood pressure
orthopedic problems (feet, back, knees)
serious falls and injuries
sleep apnea
social maladjustment
stretch marks
varicose veins
yeast infection

In addition to health problems, obese people face social barriers and discrimination and are often the object of ridicule. Obese women are less likely to marry, have less schooling, earn lower incomes, and suffer a higher rate of poverty than their thin counterparts.[5] Obese men and women are less likely to rise to the top of their careers.

The lives of obese people are daily degraded and impoverished in ways that thinner people do not experience. Morbidly obese individuals have to plan entries and exits in and out of buildings with as much care as people in wheelchairs. They must consider their girth when purchasing an automobile or choosing a seat in a restaurant. One obese patient confessed to me that since the seat belts in airplanes did not fit her, she would keep a magazine over her belly to hide the fact that she wasn't wearing one.

Finding clothes that fit and look good is a bitter challenge, yet overweight men and women have a huge assortment of clothes in their closets, which reflects all the sizes they have worn—they dare not throw out any, for who knows what gains or losses tomorrow may bring?

Obesity narrows the choice of friends. Tolerance for obesity is a litmus test for any relationship. Overweight people often shun contact with the opposite sex to avoid the pain of criticism or of being ignored. Overweight married couples may avoid sex because of the physical challenge of engaging in it. Fertility is decreased, and pregnancy is more dangerous.

Overweight people will either restrict their recreational activities to avoid embarrassment or do the opposite: push themselves into dangerous activities to prove that they can do them. I have sent more than one obese would-be marathon runner to an orthopedic surgeon. Another patient insisted on playing volleyball in college though she weighed over 300 pounds. She gave up the sport the day she saw a teammate fall on the court and be carried off by the coach and players. My patient realized that if she had been the one to fall, the entire team could not have picked her up. She gave up volleyball to spare herself the shame.

*Eighty million Americans each year "go on a diet" . . . Instead of losing weight, Americans have steadily gained weight.*

The strain of obesity on the U.S. economy is dramatic. Eighty million Americans each year "go on a diet," spending $60 billion on diet foods, books, and clinics in the process. Instead of losing weight, Americans have steadily gained weight. We are spending $32 billion a year in direct medical care for diseases caused by obesity. Many more billions are lost in destroyed lives and reduced productivity.

## When Does Excess Weight Become a Problem?

Experts disagree on the level at which obesity becomes a medical problem, but common sense dictates that it is a problem when life expectancy is reduced. The threshold level, deduced from Framingham data and life-insurance actuarial tables, is around 20 percent above ideal body weight. The life-expectancy curve slopes more steeply downward after 30 percent above ideal body weight; that level is defined as the threshold of *morbid obesity*. The ideal body weight for your gender and height can be estimated using the following formula: 100 pounds for the first 5 feet of height, plus 5 pounds for each additional inch, plus 10 pounds if you are a male. You should weigh a little less if you are young, and you may weigh a little more if you are older. I am 5'10" tall, so I should weigh 100 + (10 × 5) + 10 = 160 pounds. I actually weigh 176 pounds. I can excuse an extra 10 pounds because I am 48 years old, but the extra 6 pounds beyond that is, well, pure gravy.

Another approach is to use the Recommended Weight Ranges table shown on the following page.

### Body Mass Index: The Most Reliable Standard

The wide range in recommended weights in this table is not sufficiently precise for most scientific studies of obesity, which

**Recommended Weight Ranges for Adults[6]**

| | Weight (in pounds) | |
|---|---|---|
| Height | Women | Men |
| 4'9" | 106–118 | |
| 4'10" | 108–120 | |
| 4'11" | 110–123 | |
| 5'0" | 112–126 | |
| 5'1" | 115–129 | 126–136 |
| 5'2" | 118–132 | 128–138 |
| 5'3" | 121–135 | 130–140 |
| 5'4" | 124–138 | 132–143 |
| 5'5" | 127–141 | 134–146 |
| 5'6" | 130–144 | 137–149 |
| 5'7" | 133–147 | 140–152 |
| 5'8" | 136–150 | 143–155 |
| 5'9" | 139–153 | 146–158 |
| 5'10" | 142–156 | 149–161 |
| 5'11" | | 152–165 |
| 6'0" | | 155–169 |
| 6'1" | | 159–173 |
| 6'2" | | 162–177 |
| 6'3" | | 166–182 |

use Body Mass Index (BMI) instead. BMI is the ratio of a person's weight in kilograms to the square of that person's height in meters. BMI can be calculated using weight in pounds and height in inches by multiplying the ratio by 703.1 (rounded off to 700):

$$\text{BMI} = \frac{\text{weight in pounds} \times 700}{\text{height in inches} \times \text{height in inches}}$$

BMI is the easiest way to determine if a patient is dangerously obese, and it is the best measure to use in following the progress of weight loss.[7] Normal and abnormal ranges are as follows:

| **Body Mass Index** | |
|---|---|
| Healthy | 19–25 |
| Overweight | 26–29 |
| Morbidly obese | 30 and up |

BMI overestimates the danger for people with overdeveloped muscles—weight lifters, piano movers, and the like—but it is a pretty accurate indicator for most of us. The healthy range of BMI for women is a little higher than that for men, but not enough to require a whole new chart. Women should cluster in the 22–25 range, men 19–23. My BMI works out to 24, so I am a little heavier than I should be, the same conclusion as before.

*In 1994, 34.9 percent of U.S. adults were morbidly obese according to their Body Mass Index.*

**Percentage of Seriously Overweight People in the United States by Year and by Gender and Ethnicity**

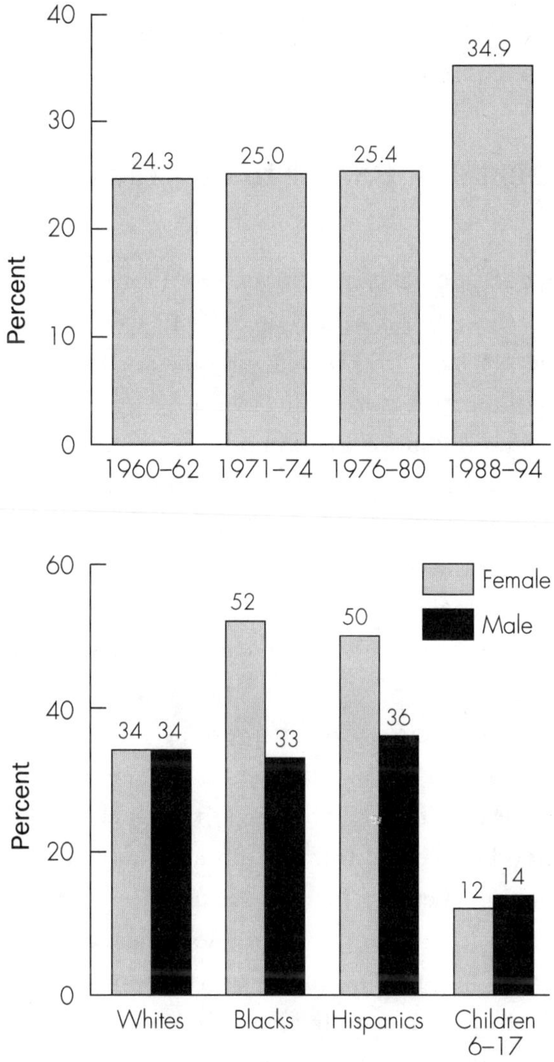


FIGURE 1.3

Between 1981 and 1991, average BMI in the United States increased from 25.3 to 26.3.[8] The increase was greatest for women, Hispanics, and African Americans, who have a national average BMI of 28.3—a serious problem. In 1994, 34.9 percent of U.S. adults were morbidly obese according to their BMI (see Figure 1.3).[9]

## Denial: A Barrier to Progress

As the saying goes, denial is not just a river in Egypt. It is a powerful defense mechanism—the one people use most often. Every day, the pleasing form of our self-image is carved out of the raw mass of our true personality by the process of blocking out that which we find unpleasant in ourselves.

Denial is not always bad; it can be constructive. In the case of obesity, it is constructive when it permits the obese patient to avoid excessive fixation on body weight and get on with an enjoyable, productive life. It is constructive when it allows a non-obese spouse to set aside any negative feelings and appreciate the obese spouse for his or her other wonderful qualities.

Denial is destructive when it prevents an obese person from admitting that obesity is a dangerous disease. It is destructive when it prevents the obese person from seeking help, or prevents a friend or partner from recommending help.

Dr. Sheldon Levine, in *The Redux Revolution,*[10] commented on how frequently physicians experience meeting a spouse or parent described as "mildly overweight" and find that the person is, in fact, massively obese. Sometimes the person underestimating the obesity used a euphemism for the sake of politeness, but more often the person who gave the faulty description honestly didn't perceive the obesity.

Doctors can overlook obesity as well. They fuss with the patient's diabetes, gout, or high blood pressure, and ignore the obvious source of the problem. In some cases they avoid discussing obesity because they believe they have no effective therapy to offer. But as new therapies such as phen-fen, Redux, and now phen-Prozac are highlighted in the media, few doctors will continue to believe that there is no effective therapy for obesity. Physicians who go on believing that their 240-pound patient is only a little overweight, who neglect to treat the obesity, are missing the chance to offer effective help. Physicians, of all people, should not engage in denial.

When normal-weight individuals worry excessively about becoming fat, or think of themselves as obese, that is a problem too. A distressing number of normal-weight people—mostly women—go to their doctors and request phen-fen or Redux prescriptions to treat self-diagnosed obesity. After performing appropriate BMI measurements, good physicians should refuse to write prescriptions, and should instead educate and reassure the patient.

The best cure for denial is an accurate weight scale and the calculated body mass index (BMI).

# Toby's Story

## PART 1

TOBY KUBILEK WEIGHED more than nine pounds when she was born. Her mother, Christina, developed diabetes during the pregnancy. Unfortunately, back then in the 1970s, doctors were less zealous in monitoring gestational diabetes. Christina had difficulty following a strict diet so Toby, typical of babies born of diabetic mothers, wound up being a very large baby, indeed. Christina had to have a cesarean section to let Toby into the world, and the rosy-skinned new baby had to remain in the intensive care unit for a few days to keep close tabs on her blood sugar. After a few anxious days, Christina and her husband, Nathan, were allowed to take their daughter home.

Toby had a normal babyhood, but by the time her brother Alex was born three years later, Toby was already showing signs of becoming overweight. At age three she weighed 38 pounds. It was not so much that she was overindulged with cookies and ice cream, but that she ate such large portions at mealtimes. In the early days, the family's friends had called Toby a cute baby and joked about her baby fat, but only Toby's mother and father laughed about her baby fat anymore. Others were too embarrassed to mention it. They could see how much weight mother and daughter had gained. Nathan stayed lean and Alex was skinny, even though the whole family ate at the same table. Christina simply reasoned that Nathan and Alex were "men" with higher rates of metabolism.

Toby was unaware that she or her mother were overweight. Weight had no meaning for her yet, but when Toby entered kindergarten, she was already 50 pounds, and she began to hear the first rumblings of societal disapproval. Some of the teachers refused to give her extra ice cream or snacks when she was still hungry, which was frequently, even though on several occasions she noticed the teachers giving extra snacks to her friends. Toby had more accidents than the other kids—knocking things over, bumping into things, often drawing disapproving looks from teachers. All kindergarten kids knock things over, but Toby, moving at high speed to keep up with the other children, had more momentum.

Nothing the teachers did, however, compared with the hurt she felt when other girls and boys started to mention her weight and call her names. Her nickname became "Tubby Toby" or "Fats." It got worse as she moved up the grades in school. Toby's mother told her to ignore the name-calling, telling her that children who called other children names were just insecure. This explanation didn't satisfy Toby because the girls calling her the names seemed to be *very* secure. They were, in fact, some of the most popular girls in the class. Toby's mother told her that these girls were rude and ill-bred, but when Toby called the offenders "rude" or "ill-bred," it didn't seem to have the same painful impact as being called "fat" or "clumsy." Toby was starting to think it might be better to be ill-bred than fat.

CHAPTER TWO

# What Causes Excess Weight Gain?

Buried deep in the brain, in a place called the hypothalamus, is the *appestat*—the appetite "thermostat." The appestat is the single most important factor in preventing excess body weight.

The existence of the appestat has been hypothesized for some time, but its significance was ignored by obesity experts until recently. In the last five years the neurology and chemistry of this important center in the brain has been more thoroughly investigated—and most obesity experts continue to ignore it. If these discoveries were made in an area other than obesity—in the field of hypertension or diabetes, for example—experts would be flocking to make use of the new information. Too many "experts" believe that obesity is about bad habits and abnormal psychology. They couldn't be more wrong.

The fundamental cause of obesity lies in the appestat. My clinical experience has taught me that most overweight people are overweight solely and simply because they are overhungry. Look at the evidence: I gave 500 patients two pills, phentermine and Prozac, told them little about diet and exercise, and many of them lost so much weight. Phentermine and Prozac produce a negligible increase in metabolism; the important effect must be the effect on the appestat.

When you think about it, we are lucky to have an appestat! Early in our evolution, human beings routinely faced starvation. Food surpluses were rare. We might have managed very well without an appestat. The human species developed powerful mechanisms to prevent weight loss, but it might not have needed a mechanism to fight weight gain.

## How the Appestat Works

When fat cells are overstuffed with fat, they produce a messenger-protein called leptin.[1] Leptin is released into the bloodstream and circulates to the appestat in the brain, where it reduces the sensation of hunger.[2] In effect, leptin tells the brain, "Stop eating, I'm full." The system is shown schematically on the right-hand side of Figure 2.1.

The details we understand at this early stage of research are enormously more complex than the picture shows.[3,4] And there is much more that we don't yet know. For instance, which neurotransmitters are involved in the leptin-appestat system? (Neurotransmitters and neuropeptides are chemical messen-

**The System That Regulates Appetite**

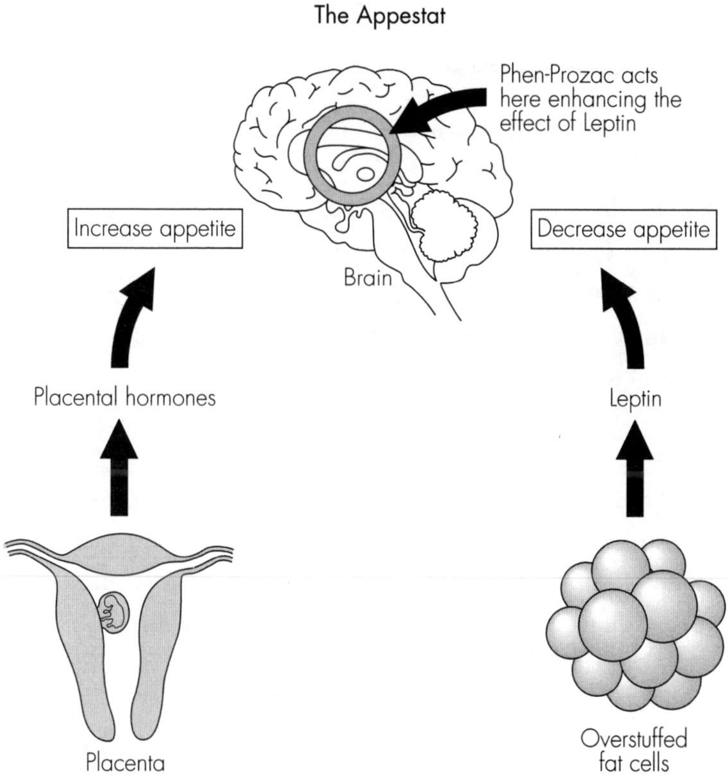


FIGURE 2.1

gers used by nerve cells to talk to each other.) Neuropeptide Y is important, because its level rises when people are starved or when they exercise. You could say that neuropeptide Y is hunger. But which neurotransmitters induce the rise in neuropeptide Y levels? It is a good bet that norepinephrine and serotonin are involved, because medications that mimic these two neurotransmitters have an effect on hunger. But it is unclear why the phen-Prozac combination suppresses the appestat so much better than either medicine alone.

## Leptin and the Appestat

When leptin was first described in 1994, researchers expected to find that obese people had a defect in the gene for leptin. They theorized that the faulty gene produced no leptin or insufficient leptin to inhibit the appestat. If this had been correct, doctors could have helped obese patients by giving them injections of leptin or developing oral drugs that mimicked the action of leptin.

To test the idea, scientists bred a strain of mice that lacked the leptin gene.[5] Given unrestricted access to food, the mice became very obese. When the mice were given injections of leptin, their appetites and weight declined to normal, as expected. Pinning hope on these promising experiments, the Amgen pharmaceutical company produced synthetic human leptin and the Eli Lilly pharmaceutical company began testing oral medicines that could mimic leptin.

Leptin itself is not useful as a treatment for ordinary obesity in humans because it has to be injected—it cannot be made into a pill—but pharmaceutical companies have been trying to produce oral medicines that mimic the action of leptin. The medicines they have developed so far, the ones that I know about, cause some weight loss, but they are not very effective because the average obese patient is already producing an excess of natural leptin; adding a little more leptin activity to an existing surplus accomplishes little.

The problem in overweight patients is that their appestat is not "listening" to leptin, and it no more listens to leptin-like drugs than it listens to naturally produced leptin. The champions of leptin hope to overcome the dullness of the appestat by creating super leptin-like drugs that will overwhelm the deaf appestat, in effect shouting at it so that it hears.

*The problem in overweight patients is that their appestat is not "listening" to leptin.*

Meanwhile, the proponents of leptin-like drugs have continued to hope that at least some obese patients will be found to be naturally deficient in leptin. Leptin-like drugs would be just the ticket for such patients. It seemed that the chemists' hopes were never going to be realized, until, in the last weeks before this book went to press, a case of naturally occuring human leptin deficiency was finally found. British researchers reported finding two obese cousins, a two-year-old boy and an eight-year-old girl, with a defect in their leptin gene.[6] They do not make active leptin. Hopefully, these two children will be helped by injections of leptin or one of the new oral leptin mimics.

Another approach to the problem of obesity is to purify and study the receptor for leptin, the protein in the appestat that binds leptin and conveys its message to the inner workings of the brain cells. The Hoffman-LaRoche company has purified the human leptin receptor. They hope to find ways to make this receptor protein work better.

I wish all these companies success in their endeavors. The physicians and pharmaceutical companies are all oarsmen in the same boat, trying to reach the same goal: to help overweight people lose excess weight. If we jostle each other along the way, claiming that one medicine is better or another approach is worse, it is only collegial bickering.

But none of these companies is likely to find a weight-loss method as cheap and effective as phen-Prozac any time soon, and phen-Prozac is already available.

## The Role of the Set-Point

The appestat model fits our everyday experience of obesity. Overweight people do not gain weight and keep on gaining, as indicated by curve A in Figure 2.2. They shift from one set-point on the appestat to a higher set-point, regulating their weight perfectly at the higher level, as shown by curve B.

It always amazed me how my 300-pound patients could eat without conscience or plan and maintain a weight consistently between 290 and 310—a 7 percent range. I eat willy-nilly too, and my weight fluctuates between 168 and 181—the same 7 percent range. It makes sense when you realize that there is a weight thermostat in the brain running the show!

There is a disease state in which the appestat appears to be missing, a rare genetic disorder called the Prader-Willi syndrome. Children with this disorder have insatiable hunger. Given free access to food, like the mice without leptin, they would literally eat themselves to death. Their weight would increase steadily without limit, as in curve A in Figure 2.2. This proves the importance of the appestat. Few children with the syndrome live into adulthood. They die young from the diseases of obesity. Recent studies in which these patients were treated with fenfluramine had partial success.[7] Treating Prader-

**Two Patterns of Weight Gain**

line A = without an appestat
line B = with an appestat

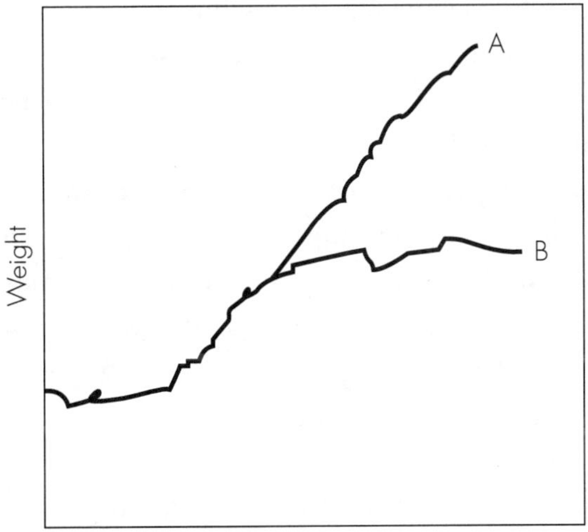


FIGURE 2.2

Willi children with phen-Prozac is a worthy concept for future studies.

## Appetite Increases During Pregnancy

The left side of Figure 2.1 is largely speculation, but there is some evidence to support it. In pregnant women the placenta produces a number of hormones that modulate the mother's metabolism for the benefit of the fetus. One hormone is human chorionic somatomammotropin (HCS); another is placental adrenocorticotropic hormone (ACTH), which induces the adrenal gland in the mother to produce more hydrocortisone. Hydrocortisone in the mother induces the mother's metabolism to convert dietary protein into fat and blocks the effect of insulin. It may soon be found that some of these hormones also increase hunger, causing the mother to eat more to support the growing fetus, which makes sense physiologically.

As any mother knows, weight gained during pregnancy can be hard to shed after delivery. The appestat can get "stuck" at the higher set-point; it may not return to its previous setting after the baby is born and the placental hormones disappear. This may have a biological purpose, since, in early humans, the extra body fat was needed to support the production of milk for the infant. I don't imagine there were many times in the life of a young cave-mother when she wasn't nursing a baby. Whatever the biological purpose, the fact has become an inconvenience for a mother who would like to get back into a size 6 after her baby is born.

## Two Kinds of Obesity

There are two kinds of obesity. Patients with *hypertrophic obesity* have the same number of fat cells as normal-weight individuals, but their fat cells are larger, being overstuffed with fat. This is the most common type of obesity and the easiest to treat. Hypertrophic patients respond well to phen-Prozac and more readily achieve ideal body weight.

The less common type of obesity is *hyperplastic obesity*. Hyperplastic individuals are born with a greater number of fat cells than their normal-weight counterparts. The main determinants are genetic. Hypertrophic people have excessive fat in the mid-body, trunk, and abdomen, but their limbs are less fat-laden. Hyperplastic people, in contrast, are fat all over. I can distinguish the two types most easily by looking at the hands. The fingers of hypertrophic people have a normal appearance; hyperplastic people have thick fingers, almost resembling sausages.

Individual fat cells in the body of a hyperplastic obese patient may not be overstuffed with fat, but the large number of fat cells gives the hyperplastic patient the appearance and all the risks of obesity. Since the individual cells in the hyperplastic patient are not overstuffed, they are individually secreting a normal amount of leptin.

For this reason, you might think that phen-Prozac would not be effective in treating hyperplastic obesity. But my experience, and the experience of other physicians, is that appetite suppressant therapy does work on hyperplastic obesity. Since there are so many more fat cells, the total of all the leptin produced is still greater than that produced in the body of a normal-weight individual. If phen-Prozac can render the appestat more sensitive to leptin, the result is still beneficial to the hyperplastic obese patient: the patient is less hungry and loses weight.

Nevertheless, the hyperplastic patient may never be able to achieve a BMI lower than 25, no matter what dose of appetite suppressant is used or how hard the patient tries to diet. I think this is because, after some weight has been lost, leptin production by the fat cells is turned off. Further improvement in the sensitivity of the appestat is then useless.

## Excess Weight Loss

Our appetite for food is not a single monolithic drive, solely determined by the current setting of the appestat. Appetite is a complex mixture of psychology, biochemistry, personality, and willpower. Until recently, psychologists, dietitians, and physicians have behaved as though appetite were only a matter of psychology.

---

*Appetite is a complex mixture of psychology, biochemistry, personality, and willpower.*

---

To illustrate what an oversimplification that is, let's consider anorexia nervosa. Most common in girls in countries where female slenderness is held in high esteem, "anorexia" would seem to be clearly a disease of abnormal psychology.

Anorexics perceive themselves to be fat even after they become dangerously thin as a result of undereating. Their menstrual periods stop. Their mental acuity declines. These girls are, in fact, starving. Are they hungry? They must be in some sense, but the powerful psychological overlay—the abnormal perception of body image—overwhelms their physical sense of hunger.

When scientists start to look at the appestat in anorexics, they will likely find that the structure of the appestat is normal. Many anorexics will be found to be depressed. In fact, Prozac was discovered because of a biochemical link between depression and bulimia, a disorder related to anorexia (see page 36). But not all anorexics suffer from depression, just as most patients with depression are not anorexic.

## Why Phen-Prozac Won't Cause Excess Weight Loss

When I first learned about phen-fen, I worried that anorexics would use it to lose weight and do themselves harm. I no longer worry about this, because neither phen-fen nor phen-Prozac work on the normal component of appetite; they work only on the abnormal component. Before I understood this I gave phen-Prozac to two young models who each weighed about 120 pounds. They believed they would do better in their careers if they weighed 110 pounds. I calculated that they would remain within the 19–25 BMI range even if they lost 10 pounds. I did not give them phen-fen because of the PPH risk it carries, but I was willing to give them phen-Prozac. However, it didn't work; the models didn't lose weight.[8] I know of other doctors who have given phen-fen to women of similar weight, and those women did not lose weight either.

Anorexics would not be at risk to lose more weight on a phen-Prozac program. Since they already weigh below ideal body weight, there is no abnormal component of appetite for phen-Prozac to work on. Actually, the Prozac in the combination might work out to be helpful for anorexics. Ongoing studies have in fact shown that many anorexics benefit from taking an antidepressant such as Prozac. Whether this is because depression is co-existing with anorexia nervosa, or the antidepressant has a specific, beneficial effect on anorexia nervosa itself is unknown.

I also used to worry that if I didn't closely follow patients as they approached ideal body weight on the phen-Prozac program, they might go past the point of ideal weight and keep going into the range of unhealthy low weight (see Figure 2.3).

**Two Patterns of Weight Loss**

IBW stands for Ideal Body Weight. The bars represent total hunger. The shaded portions of the bars represent the abnormal component of hunger. Line B represents the pattern of weight loss experienced by patients on phen-Prozac. Line A represents a hypothetical pattern of unchecked weight loss.

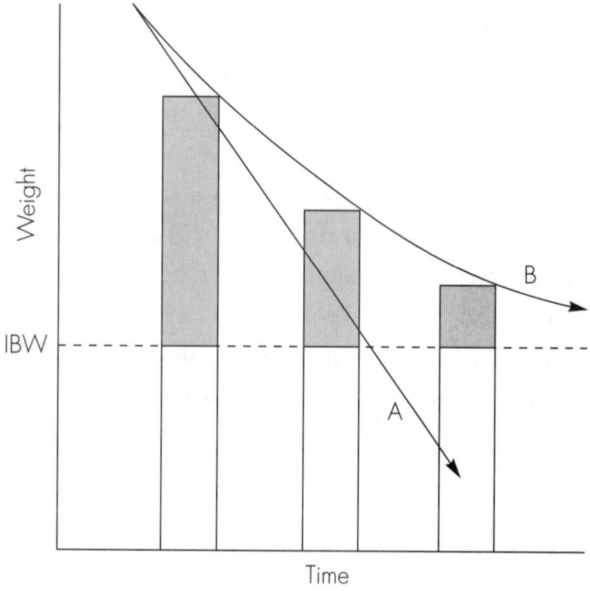


FIGURE 2.3

I need not have worried. None of my patients on a phen-Prozac weight loss program went below their ideal body weight, no matter how infrequently we had office visits. Phen-Prozac and phen-fen act only on the abnormal part of appetite. This abnormal component is depicted as shaded bars in the graph in Figure 2.3. Notice how the bars get shorter as the person approaches ideal body weight. Treating very obese individuals can therefore be easier than treating those with only a little weight to lose.

## Can Hunger Be Controlled by Will?

If people with diseases such as anorexia nervosa can learn to suppress hunger pangs through psychology, why shouldn't normal overweight people be able to learn how to suppress their hunger through an act of willpower? Why can't they lose weight—without medication—by exercising self-control?

Some people can. Voluntary dieting does sometimes succeed as a permanent solution for obesity. If you are overweight and can ignore or suppress your appetite by an act of will, do it! If a psychotherapist, dietitian, your mother, Robert Atkins, or your spiritual counselor can help you take control of your appetite and habits, you won't need a phen-Prozac program. Statistics show, however, that it is the rare person who can successfully lose weight and keep it off using willpower alone.

*Statistics show that it is the rare person who can successfully lose weight and keep it off using willpower alone.*

# Toby's Story

## PART 2

LIKE MOST SEVEN- and eight-year-old girls, Toby loved dolls. But it didn't help her self-image that her Barbie dolls had waists like wasps. The girls in the Disney cartoons were all shaped like Barbie. Fat people were ridiculed on TV sitcoms. Even at her young age, Toby saw the world's insensitivity toward overweight people. Alex, her younger brother, was cruel to Toby, often teasing her about being his *big* sister; of course, that was to be expected from a younger brother. She could always beat him up and put an end to his sniping for a few days, but it irked her that Alex stayed so thin. She wondered how he could eat candy and cookies whenever he pleased and never get fat.

When Toby entered sixth grade, she weighed over 120 pounds and was developing breasts. Her mother had been a little precocious, too. The early development was a bit of an embarrassment to Toby because she had been trying to avoid attention. She wore oversized, sloppy T-shirts every day to hide her new curves. She was a good student, bright and conscientious. She was very close to several of her teachers, who now tried to protect her from some of the ridicule she endured. Toby's parents consulted a doctor at this point about her weight and precocious puberty. The doctor told them that her sexual development was early but within normal limits. As for the weight, he could only suggest placing her on a low-fat diet. He did not want to emphasize diet too much, for fear of inhibiting her vertical growth and causing her to obsess about her body, which might lead to eating disorders later.

By now Toby was aware that her mother was overweight. As Toby developed a sense of who she was, she became painfully conscious of who her mother was also. It didn't help that at about that time her mother developed full-fledged diabetes. There were always bottles of diabetes pills in the bathroom, packets of artificial sweetener on the table, and diet foods in the pantry. Christina was always talking about her diet and how deprived she felt from its restrictions. Toby often felt confused by her mother's attitude toward food. At times Christina withheld food from Toby to prevent her further weight gain; other times she seemed to lavish food on her family—apparently getting vicarious pleasure from watching them eat the food she couldn't. Christina jogged around the neighborhood several days a week wearing a sweatshirt and Spandex pants. Toby was very embarrassed about it.

Toby's father was constantly reminding her to do more exercise. She preferred to exercise secretly, but she had trouble sticking to any program. She didn't participate much in gym at school, because she did not want to be seen. She was left out of sports altogether because she was so uncoordinated. Her mother suggested a dance class, but after one look at herself in the mirror standing next to the other willowy girls, Toby wanted no part of it. She cried silently the whole way home.

CHAPTER THREE

# The Phen–Fenomenon

To understand how and why phen-Prozac was developed, we first must look at the histories of such drugs as Pondimin, Redux, and phen-fen. These weight-loss therapies, developed in the 1970s and 1980s, broke new ground in the medical treatment of obesity and paved the way for phen-Prozac.

## Development of Fenfluramine

Fenfluramine gained attention in the early 1970s when scientists noted a relationship between the levels of serotonin in the brain and an eating disorder called bulimia.[1] Serotonin, a naturally occurring neurotransmitter, is involved in the brain centers associated with sleep, feelings of well-being, sex drive, and appetite. Bulimic patients, mostly young women, alternate between eating large amounts of fattening food and purging themselves by vomiting. Scientists found that bulimic women had low levels of serotonin in their brains.

Bulimics were known to be prone to depression. This led scientists at the pharmaceutical company Eli Lilly to suspect that low serotonin levels might have something to do with depression. Depression got most of the attention after that, because a lot more people suffer from depression than from bulimia. The Eli Lilly company looked at a large number of compounds that could increase serotonin levels in the brain, including fenfluramine, which had been recently synthesized by the Orsem-Servier company in France. Fenfluramine had several drawbacks as a treatment for depression, however: it had to be taken several times a day and caused a number of undesirable side effects.

Eli Lilly looked at many other compounds similar to fenfluramine and ultimately discovered Prozac. In clinical trials, Prozac taken once a day was very effective in treating depression and had fewer side effects than fenfluramine. Some patients in the open trial of Prozac were noted to lose weight, which was regarded as a nuisance side effect by researchers and not immediately followed up.

## The Wurtmans' Pioneering Weight-Loss Research

In the early 1970s, Richard Wurtman, M.D., a neurologist at MIT, was looking at fenfluramine in a different context. Dr. Wurtman and his wife Judy, a nutritionist, had been interested in finding a better treatment for obesity. They had noticed that many of the foods obese patients prefer, such as dairy desserts and fatty meats, were high in proteins containing the amino acid tryptophan. Tryptophan eaten in large quantities raises the levels of serotonin in the brain. It occurred to the Wurtmans that overweight people might be using high-tryptophan foods as drugs, inducing a sense of well-being by raising brain serotonin levels.[2] The fact that high-tryptophan foods were also fattening foods led to the obesity. If a medicine could be found to raise the serotonin level, perhaps overweight people would find it easier to give up favorite fattening foods.

The Wurtmans formed a company called Interneuron and obtained the U.S. rights to fenfluramine. In tests, the drug proved modestly effective as a weight-loss agent, but it caused diarrhea and drowsiness in many patients. Interneuron obtained FDA approval for the use of fenfluramine in treating obesity and named the drug Pondimin. The Wurtmans licensed Pondimin to the A. H. Robins Company, which was then at the zenith of its marketing power.

Pondimin did not sell well; doctors were still skittish about using drugs to treat obesity. Then the A. H. Robins Company was slammed with a massive class-action suit by women who had suffered damage from an unrelated product, the Dalkon Shield. Robins was not eager to promote any more controversial products. Pondimin languished on the shelf.

Dr. Wurtman realized that sales of Pondimin would have been stalled even with a more eager vendor. A way had to be found to reduce the side effects of Pondimin.

## Redux to the Rescue?

At the request of Dr. Wurtman, chemists at Orsem-Servier in France were striving to make Pondimin work better. The chemists knew the fenfluramine molecule exists in two distinct forms that are mirror images of each other: the right-handed isomer (dexfenfluramine) and the left-handed isomer (levo-fenfluramine). Such forms are called *stereoisomers.* Pondimin is an equal mixture of the two isomers. The chemists found a way to make pure dexfenfluramine.

Biological systems usually interact with only one isomer of a drug, and the appetite center in the brain is no exception. Only dexfenfluramine has any significant effect on the appestat, and it causes fewer side effects. The levo form contributes nothing but the drowsiness and diarrhea mentioned earlier.

The Wurtmans obtained the U.S. rights to the new preparation of pure dexfenfluramine and named it Redux. Interneuron and Orsem-Servier mounted a heavy push to get the FDA to approve Redux for sale in the United States, a story that's told in detail in Chapter 4.

However, hopes for Redux may have been too high. Because Pondimin never worked that well, why would Redux work so much better? After all, Pondimin and Redux have the same chemical formula (see Appendix). Redux might have fewer side effects than Pondimin, but why would it be more effective? It is nothing more than the dextro-isomer of a drug in which we were already disappointed. In one head-to-head study, Redux was no more effective than Pondimin.[3] Meanwhile, the search for other medical weight-loss therapies was continuing elsewhere.

## Phen-Fen Enters the Scene

Phen-fen was the brainchild of Michael Weintraub, M.D., a physician-scientist at the University of Rochester School of

Medicine in New York, in the early 1980s. He was aware that the U.S. population, after a period of fastidiousness and improving health in the 1970s, was forgetting all about fat and calories, embarking on a national eating spree that increased the national average body weight by eight pounds.[4] One-third of all Americans were obese, by the usual standard of being 20 percent above their ideal body weight. Many were morbidly obese—30 percent above ideal body weight. There was ample evidence that obesity was at least as dangerous as high blood pressure in causing heart attacks and strokes, and that it increased the risk of cancer as well.[5] Something had to be done!

Short-term studies using single appetite suppressants had met with little success, and non-medical programs employing diet and exercise alone were notoriously prone to failure. The majority of individuals who lost weight in programs such as Weight Watchers, Jenny Craig, and Physicians Weight-Loss Center gained all the weight back after leaving the program. Dr. Weintraub decided to undertake a study where the subjects used everything at once—diet and exercise and multiple medications—to see how much weight loss could be achieved using maximal therapy. He pulled out all the stops, giving patients both phentermine and fenfluramine. This was the first of his original ideas.

His second original idea was to extend the study beyond the six weeks observed in previous studies of appetite suppressant drugs. Doctors had worried that appetite suppressants might be addictive or cause harmful long-term effects. There was no evidence of such effects in studies at the time, but physicians worried nevertheless because the available appetite suppressants were chemically related to other, older medicines, such as Dexedrine, that were known to have harmful effects.

The prevailing belief before Dr. Weintraub's study was that the causes of obesity were behavioral and psychological. Behavior modification and psychoanalysis were recognized as the high road to obesity therapy; drug therapy was frowned upon.

Dr. Weintraub disagreed with this narrow way of thinking. He wrote:

> Both the medical profession and society look with disfavor on obese people and obesity in general. For example, students at a well-known university preferred a number of less savory people to obese individuals as marriage partners. Obese people are treated negatively in cartoons and in literature. Many believe that obese people need only to "close their mouths" and to be more motivated to lose weight. Thus, use of medications to correct a characterologic defect is, in the opinion of physicians and the public, deemed inappropriate.[6]

When appetite suppressant drugs were used to treat obesity, the standard practice was to prescribe them for only two to six weeks, in conjunction with diet and exercise. As soon as the patient started to achieve success, the medicines were discontinued. Dr. Weintraub remarked wryly: "The [appetite suppressant] drugs were the only drugs physicians expected to continue working after they were discontinued."[7] He noted that no one discontinued blood pressure medicines after six weeks, fearing that the patient might become dependent on them. No one cared whether diabetics were "addicted" to insulin. Only appetite suppressants were singled out for discrimination. Dr. Weintraub was determined to free himself from that prejudice.

### First Double-Blind Study of Phen-Fen

Dr. Weintraub's experiment was performed as a double-blind study, the most reliable format. In a double-blind study, neither the patients nor the doctor know whether medicine or placebo is being administered to a given individual. This design assures that any variation in results is attributable to the medicines, not to the biases of the investigators or the patients.

The double-blind phase of Dr. Weintraub's study lasted thirty-five weeks. This phase was followed by a two-year open-label phase, during which all the patients remaining in the study continued their regimen of phentermine and fenfluramine. The purpose of this phase was to find out if any harmful effects accrued from long-term use, and to see if the weight loss achieved during the first part of the study could be maintained.

The study initially involved 121 patients. Their average age was forty, and their average weight was 202 pounds. Seventy-five percent of the participants were women. This was a fair representation of the portion of the U.S. population that was at greatest risk for obesity. All of the patients received counseling in diet and exercise, and there were regular checkups to determine that they were following a low-fat diet, exercising, and taking the medication.

When the study was completed after two years, Dr. Weintraub found that, almost without exception, the patients taking phentermine and fenfluramine lost weight—thirty-one pounds on average—and kept the weight off as long as they took the medicines. The patients who received a placebo lost a little weight at first, but gained the weight back by the end of the double-blind phase of the study. Rarely in medicine are results as clear-cut as they are in the main graph from the study (see Figure 3.1).

**Dr. Weintraub's Experiment**

One hundred twenty-one obese subjects on phen-fen vs. placebo

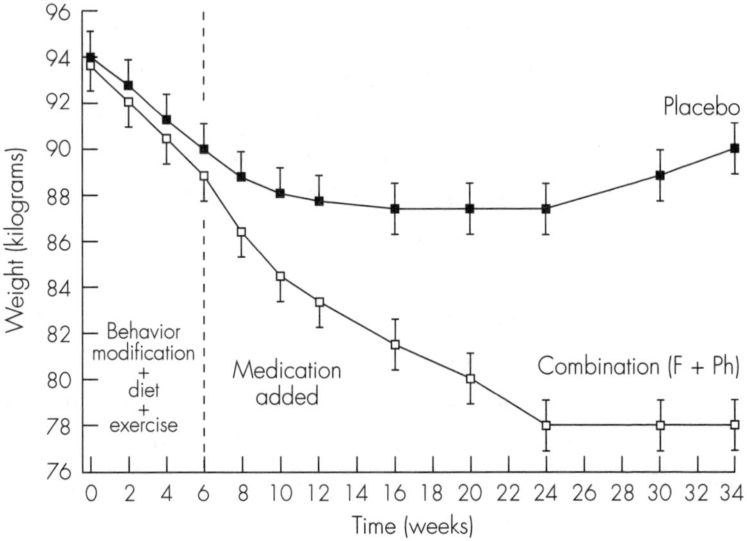


FIGURE 3.1

Dr. Weintraub observed that there seemed to be a leveling off of the weight loss after thirty weeks; the early rate of rapid weight loss was not sustained. I have heard some lecturers, including Dr. Weintraub himself, speak of this leveling off as though it were a problem with the therapy. But Dr. Weintraub's patients were 202 pounds at the start; by thirty weeks, after losing one to two pounds per week, they were approaching their ideal body weight. We don't need a therapy that will work any better than that! All the patients lost enough weight to restore their risk of death and disease to normal, and none of them gained the weight back so long as they took the medicines.

## News of Phen-Fen Spreads

The tidal wave Dr. Weintraub set in motion gathered speed. In my home state of Maryland, Dr. Gabe Mirkin, host of a national radio talk show, promoted the treatment on his daily radio program. He appreciated the significance of Dr. Weintraub's discovery immediately and began prescribing phen-fen to his obese patients; he has treated thousands by now. Dr. Richard Rothman, a noted psychiatrist and research psychopharmacologist, opened the Be-Lite Medical Centers in Largo, Maryland, and north Virginia. Dr. Mark Eig of Silver Spring, Maryland, and other physicians in my area learned about phen-fen through medical journals, newspapers, and rumors, and started to prescribe it cautiously. Dr. Peter Hitzig set up a Web site to dispense information to the public and obtained a trademark on the name "fen-phen." Dr. Sheldon Levine in New Jersey and Dr. Michael Steelman in Oklahoma prescribed phen-fen successfully to thousands of obese patients. Dr. Steven Lamm in Utah prescribed phen-fen to patients, and along with Gerald Couzens, wrote an excellent book about phen-fen entitled *Thinner at Last* (Simon & Schuster, 1995, 1996).

But acceptance was far from universal. In many states, the use of appetite suppressants beyond six weeks was discouraged by state medical boards; in other states, it was outright illegal. Some physicians were prosecuted for prescribing long-term appetite suppressants. The threat of malpractice suits hung over every physician's head. Any departure from the traditional standard of care, no matter how promising, is regarded as a target of opportunity for malpractice attorneys.

A phen-fen underground developed. Physicians continued to prescribe the medicines, because they were so clearly effective and there was little else to offer obese patients. Physicians knew the serious health risks obese patients faced, and most physicians had consistently dismal results with voluntary diet programs.

In 1995, Dr. Richard Atkinson and his colleagues at the University of Wisconsin published an open trial of phen-fen with 467 patients in an office practice setting, followed over a period of nine months.[8] Their patients lost an average of 37.4 pounds over the course of the study. Twenty-seven dropped out because of relatively minor side effects such as insomnia, nervousness, nausea, and heart palpitations. It was significant that both blood pressure and cholesterol levels dropped among the study patients. My colleagues, Drs. Eig and Rothman, and I have confirmed this finding. It was reasonable to monitor phentermine, a stimulant, to see if it would increase the systemic blood pressure, but that concern has proved unfounded. Data have shown that phen-fen and phen-Prozac can be used in patients with moderately high blood pressure.[9] By 1996, Dr. Atkinson had extended his study to 1,347 subjects with the same reassuring results.[10]

The word about phen-fen gradually reached the news media. In March of 1994, Dr. Weintraub's picture appeared in *The Washingtonian* magazine, in an article entitled "Keep It Off." The doctor and his program appeared again in a sidebar to the cover story "Fat Times" in *Time* magazine in January of 1995. There were articles in *Woman's Day* (April 1995), *U.S. News & World Report* (May 1995), and *Reader's Digest* (April 1996). In March of 1995, Dr. Weintraub and six of his study participants discussed phen-fen with Hugh Downs on *20/20.*

Thousands of physicians across the country started prescribing phen-fen to millions of obese patients, with amazing success. Perhaps as significant as the weight loss itself is the fact that physicians and patients and the public were awakened to a new understanding: obesity is not merely about diet and habits, but results from a specific chemical disorder in the brain, for which effective chemical responses now exist.

*Obesity is not merely about diet and habits, but results from a specific chemical disorder in the brain.*

Phen-fen seemed to be the perfect solution for treating obesity, but a serious flaw was discovered: fenfluramine is strongly linked with a lung disorder called primary pulmonary hypertension, which we'll examine next.

# Toby's Story

**PART 3**

TOBY FIRST BEGAN TO NOTICE boys in the sixth grade. The boys first began to notice her a year later. At first, this development brought her great happiness. She even considered joining the dance class when she found out some of the boys were in the class. But it seemed that whenever she felt a little hope, her extra weight brought her back to reality. Soon the "pairing off" of couples started in her class. Although the boys were taller now, Toby was still conscious of how much bigger she was. She was afraid that if she joined the dance class, the boys would notice the rolls of fat when they put their arms around her waist. They would not be able to pick her up and swing her the way they did the slender girls. She would always feel self-conscious and be on the defensive.

All of the television shows and movies and magazines stressed the importance of romance. Toby read *Seventeen* magazine, even though she was a few years shy of seventeen. She read all about dating and sexual matters, and she was worried about her future. She could see the difference between herself and her thin friends, as well as the models in *Seventeen* magazine. She wondered if a fat girl would ever experience the same love and romance that seemed to come so naturally to all the skinny girls. She had many serious conversations with her mother and her best friend Bonny, about how she could get into the social scene at school. But Toby was painfully aware that, especially for teenagers, "thin was in" and she wasn't.

She decided that the "quiet, good student" approach would no longer work. She was being ignored by her peers and was starved for some affection. Instead, she thrust herself into the limelight. She went to many parties whether invited or not. She decided to be more outgoing and had a few parties of her own. She was a good talker and she knew it, and she tried hard to be a trustworthy friend. These were all good developments.

Before long she had some close girlfriends and a few boy "buddies," but no real boyfriend. She felt she was on the verge. She had lost some weight by nearly starving herself—for a month she had tried to drink only fruit juice, but she had felt miserable.

Andy, an overweight boy in the class, kept trying to get her attention, but she ignored him. She knew that if she linked up with him, she would never escape the trap. She didn't want to be reminded of her weight problem. She wanted a slender boyfriend, like Bonny's or Judy's.

Tim Stanwich took Toby to the senior prom. She couldn't believe her good luck. She had felt resigned to not have a date, but Tim asked her out. He was a nice, intelligent boy. He treated her respectfully and seemed to enjoy her fun personality. She was embarrassed that she sweated so much dancing with him. She wished, too, that she had taken the dance classes. When Tim tried to twirl her, she stumbled awkwardly and split her dress in the back.

They went out a few more times after that, but Tim began to get on her nerves. It annoyed her that whenever they sat in the back of a car, Tim would pat her affectionately on the side of her legs. She thought he was trying to call attention to her fat thighs. She knew better, but she couldn't stop thinking it. Later, Bonny confessed to her a conversation she had overheard between her boyfriend and Tim, in which Tim had said he hoped Toby would "put out" for him soon, because she was so fat and couldn't get a boyfriend any other way. Toby felt bruised and shattered inside. She never answered Tim's phone calls after that.

CHAPTER FOUR

# Fenfluramine's Fatal Flaw

The good news that obesity is a chemical disorder and can be treated with medications such as phen-fen was followed by bad news: fenfluramine in both its commercial forms, Pondimin and Redux, has been shown to cause primary pulmonary hypertension (PPH) in some people.[1] Primary pulmonary hypertension is a disease in which the blood vessels in the lungs are inexorably destroyed, causing the lung to fail as a gas-exchanger. The first symptom of PPH is shortness of breath.[2] At first, the patient is short of breath only as a result of exercise, but as the disease progresses the patient becomes short of breath even when at rest. In later stages, there is chest pain with breathing, the patient feels tired and weak, and supplemental oxygen is of little use. It makes little difference how much oxygen is in the lungs if there are no blood vessels to pick it up. In advanced stages, patients may pass out and cough up blood.

Under normal circumstances, all the blood pumped out of the right side of the heart into the pulmonary artery must traverse the lungs to reach the left side of the heart. The pressure in the pulmonary artery is normally low because the normal lung is so rich in large blood vessels; it is easy to pump blood through the normal lung. When blood vessels in the lung become reduced and constricted by PPH, pressure rises in the pulmonary artery. The walls of the right side of the heart thicken to sustain the increased burden of pumping.

Blood may leak through the *foramen ovale,* a flap connection between the right and left side of the heart. When the pressure in the right side of the heart rises sufficiently, the foramen ovale opens, allowing blood to bypass the lung altogether. That takes some of the strain off the right side of the heart, but the blood pumped into the left side lacks oxygen, having bypassed the lung. The patient's lips, hands, and feet turn blue. This ugly sequence of events is called *cor pulmonale.* Death is not far off when this develops. The patient may die of asphyxiation, acidosis (acid in the blood), or a heart attack.

Of all patients with PPH, half die within the first two years after diagnosis is made. A few patients who contract PPH from fenfluramine are able to return to normal if the disease is caught early and fenfluramine use is discontinued,[3] but most patients die or are permanently crippled. Medicines called calcium-channel blockers help some patients, but they are not a sure bet. Many patients can be saved only by a heart-lung transplant; you can imagine the complexity and risk of such surgery.

**The Heart and Lungs in Normal Subjects and in Patients with PPH**

RV = right ventricle PA = pulmonary artery PV = pulmonary vein

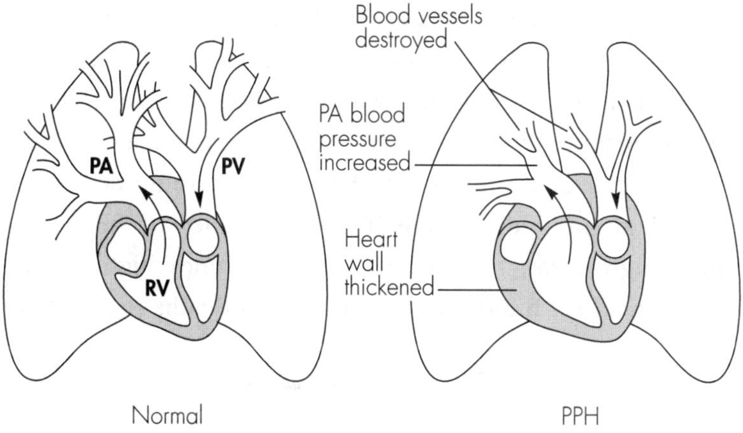


FIGURE 4.1

You know that PPH is a serious disease when a heart-lung transplant is the recommended treatment!

After a heart-lung transplant, if the patient survives the surgery—a big "if"—the patient must be maintained on medication to suppress the immune system to prevent rejection of the transplanted heart and lung. Many patients die of infections or cancer that can develop as a result of the immunosuppression.

## Prevalence of PPH

PPH is not a common disease.[4] It is difficult to measure how common it is, but it has become important to ascertain its frequency in the general population because we know that fenfluramine and Redux increase the frequency of PPH about thirty times.[5] The increased risk of PPH from fenfluramine use would not be as worrisome if the frequency of PPH in the general population were only two in one million, as the Wyeth-Ayerst company, maker of Redux, claims. Using that figure, we would expect to see sixty cases of PPH per one million patients on fenfluramine. Although the possibility of sixty deaths out of one million fenflurmine users is troubling, consider that the remaining 999,940 patients could be saved from death and the diseases associated with obesity. However, we would be terribly worried about fenfluramine if the frequency of PPH were much higher, say, ten or one hundred times higher. That would mean six hundred or six thousand deaths per million.

*PPH is not a common disease . . . [but] we know that fenfluramine and Redux increase the frequency of PPH about thirty times.*

In 1996, the first year many physicians were aware of phen-fen and Redux, six million new prescriptions were written for phen-fen, and three million for Redux. There were eighteen million total prescriptions for phen-fen, so each patient on phen-fen refilled the prescription an average of three times. Since the average prescription for phen-fen was for one month, that means the average patient on phen-fen took the medicines for longer than three months. That is important, since Dr. Abenhaim of McGill University in Montreal showed that the risk of PPH from fenfluramine goes up after three months of use. Even with the conservative figure of two cases of PPH per million on fenfluramine, the current rate of use would amount to 360 new cases of PPH per year. The *CBS Nightly News,* on May 5, 1997, reported the death of a young Massachusetts woman who was taking phen-fen. The reporter correctly observed that there have been no reported instances of PPH with phentermine alone in the thirty years of its use, making fenfluramine the likely culprit. *All Things Considered,* on public radio on May 15, 1997, reported that the National Institutes of Health (NIH) has been following a "dozen" cases of PPH associated with fenfluramine.

Skeptics could argue that the young woman's death might have been a chance association between PPH and fenfluramine. PPH does occur, rarely, in people who do not take fenfluramine. Perhaps the woman in Massachusetts would have developed PPH even if she had not taken fenfluramine. A malpractice suit has been lodged by the woman's family against the doctor and the Wyeth-Ayerst company, and a jury will have to decide.

PPH is a difficult disease to diagnose. Many physicians are not even aware of its existence. The symptoms of PPH, shortness of breath and chest pain, are often diagnosed as other, more common diseases. Few patients who die of undiagnosed PPH have an autopsy. Even when PPH is recognized, the disease is seldom reported to the Centers for Disease Control in Atlanta (CDC) or the NIH. If there were a burgeoning epidemic of PPH in the United States as a result of increased fenfluramine use, we might not know about it.

You have to ask whether the "iceberg" under the fenfluramine-PPH "tip" is a true iceberg or just an ice cube. Unfortunately, there is reason to believe it's a real iceberg.

The PPH registry at the Centers for Disease Control found 187 cases of PPH in data collected from thirty-two centers between 1981 and 1985. Rich and Brundage[6] found PPH at autopsy in 1 percent of patients in whom the right side of heart was enlarged. Walcott and colleagues[7] found twenty-three cases in the records of the Mayo Clinic from 1946 to 1965. Such data are interesting; the statistics confirm that the disease is rare, but they don't give us a precise handle on the frequency because they don't tell us the total number of cases out of which the described number of PPH cases was seen.

A review of 17,901 autopsies performed at Johns Hopkins University Hospital from 1944 to 1965 yielded twenty-four cases of PPH.[8] That translates into a prevalence of 0.13 percent in the population—thirteen hundred per million, not the two per million claimed by proponents of Redux. If this high frequency is accurate, we have a scary situation.

PPH affects women more often than men, young women more often than older women. The majority of people using Redux or phen-fen are young women, so it is less reassuring that PPH is rare in the general population. It is not fair to use the whole population as the basis for calculating the frequency of PPH, if only a subgroup of the population is really at risk. If the twenty-four cases of PPH seen in the Johns Hopkins autopsy study were divided by the number of young women in the group (surely a small fraction!) instead of by the total number of autopsies (17,901), a much higher frequency of PPH would result.

I have reviewed the literature to find the source of the two-per-million figure used by Wyeth-Ayerst in defending Redux to physicians, but have not been able to find the source of that statistic. The Products Services Department at Wyeth-Ayerst has informed me that the figure was taken from prepublication data provided by Dr. Lucien Abenhaim, based on statistics of patients in Belgium. Dr. Abenhaim and his colleagues in other European countries published their summary article in the *New England Journal of Medicine* in August 1996.[9] The article does not mention any specific frequency of PPH in the background population; it says only that the disease is rare.

I'm not saying that the two-in-a-million figure is wrong. It might be correct. Thirteen hundred per million may be right, too. We just don't know for certain what the frequency of PPH in the population is, but there is a lot riding on the answer and we must monitor the situation closely.

## Aminorex and Spanish Oil: Evidence That PPH Can Be Caused by Drugs

Several localized outbreaks of PPH in Europe have occurred in the past, traceable to a new drug or a contaminated food product. There was an outbreak in Spain in 1983, after a large number of people ingested rapeseed oil contaminated with aniline and acetanilide dyes.[10] Most patients died quickly from pulmonary edema, but survivors developed PPH. This shows that it is not unreasonable to think that drugs can cause PPH.

Between 1967 and 1970, there was a twentyfold rise in incidence of PPH in Switzerland, Austria, and Germany after the introduction of a new appetite suppressant, Aminorex.[11,12] One person in a thousand who took Aminorex developed PPH. *One in a thousand, not one in a million.* After Aminorex was withdrawn from the market, the prevalence of PPH diminished.

PPH was also seen in some users of phenformin,[13] a diabetes medicine taken off the market in the seventies because it produced lactic acidosis, a serious condition in which the blood is acidified. If fenfluramine really does cause PPH, it would not be the first drug to do so.

### Why Fenfluramine Causes PPH

There is early evidence that fenfluramine causes PPH by releasing serotonin in the blood. Serotonin is a neurotransmitter in the brain, and it is naturally present in many other parts of the body. The cells that surround blood vessels produce serotonin and secrete it into the blood. Serotonin is a potent vasoconstrictor; it causes the muscular walls of arteries to contract, restricting blood flow. The arteries would be constricted all the time, except that serotonin in blood plasma is sucked into platelets as rapidly as it is made. Platelets are the little cells in blood responsible for stopping blood flow from cuts and wounds. Platelets take up serotonin and store it for emergency use. When you have a bleeding cut, the wound is initially plugged up with a clump of platelets—like using egg yolks to stop a leak in a radiator. The platelets in the clump release substances that cause the formation of a blood clot at the site, plus they release serotonin to reduce the blood flow to the cut, slowing the blood loss. It is an excellent system.

In the millions of people on phen-fen and Redux, fenfluramine causes platelets to release stored serotonin into the blood plasma and prevents the platelets from taking the serotonin back up again.[14] The level of serotonin in the blood plasma increases significantly. This fact was only recently discovered and its consequences are unclear, but it is tempting to speculate that mobilization of platelet serotonin has a lot to do with the development of fenfluramine-associated PPH. In PPH, the blood vessels in the lung are constricted to the point that they are obliterated. The loss of so many blood vessels from the lung causes high blood pressure in the remaining vessels, hence pulmonary hypertension.

But why doesn't everyone taking fenfluramine develop PPH? Why only a few people? Obviously, there is more to learn.

It is not a settled issue that PPH is caused by increased serotonin in the blood. There are, in fact, several competing hypotheses regarding the cause of PPH. Another prominent hypothesis is that fenfluramine blocks the potassium current in pulmonary artery muscle cells, causing chronic constriction of the pulmonary arteries.[15] Dr. Kenneth Weir has shown this to be true in isolated artery-muscle cells in the laboratory. He is currently testing phentermine and Prozac to see if they, too, affect the potassium current. The results will not be available by the time this book goes to press, but I suspect he will find that they do not significantly affect the potassium current at normal doses, since neither Prozac nor phentermine has been statistically associated with PPH. Fenfluramine and Aminorex were extremely potent inhibitors of the potassium current.

On the other hand, it may well be that the increased serotonin in blood is the cause of fenfluramine-induced PPH; Dr. Weir's experiments do not exclude this explanation. Some experts have claimed that the absence of any reported association between PPH and carcinoid syndrome is evidence against the serotonin hypothesis, but this argument is extremely weak. Carcinoid cancer is a form of colon cancer in which the cancer cells secrete large amounts of serotonin into the bloodstream. The extra serotonin is known to cause deleterious changes in the heart valves, but carcinoid cancer is not known to cause PPH. However, since carcinoid is rare and PPH is rare, I doubt that any association between the two will ever be seen, even if it exists.

However, we now have a large number of people taking fenfluramine. If increased serotonin in the blood really is the cause of fenfluramine-induced PPH—and I believe that it is—then we can confidently predict that a number of cases of fenfluramine-associated heart valve disease will be discovered in the near future.

## Why Prozac Does Not Cause PPH

I'll cover more about Prozac in the next chapter, but let me explain now that Prozac does not release serotonin from platelets; it works by a different mechanism than fenfluramine. Fenfluramine releases serotonin from most tissues that store it. Prozac only blocks the reabsorption system in the brain. There is no reason to think that Prozac affects platelets in the blood. In addition, Prozac is more than 98 percent protein-bound in the blood; very little is free to have an effect on blood cells. Fenfluramine is much less protein-bound, so more is available to cause trouble.

---

> *It is apparent that Prozac has not increased the frequency of PPH in the ten years it has been in use.*

---

When we consider the mechanisms by which fenfluramine and Prozac work, we do not expect an association between Prozac and PPH, and none has been seen! The Eli Lilly company has been tracking the frequency of all side effects and adverse events associated with Prozac since it was approved in the United States and Europe in 1987. Since then, out of nineteen million patients taking Prozac worldwide, eight cases of PPH have been reported. Using the lowest estimate of the background frequency of PPH in the general population (two per million), thirty-eight cases would have been expected. Even allowing for underreporting of PPH, it is apparent that Prozac has not increased the frequency of PPH in the ten years it has been in use.

In contrast, in 1996, the first year that Redux and Pondimin were in frequent use in the United States, twenty-two cases of fenfluramine-associated PPH were reported to the NIH, with more probably on the way.

## Why Did the FDA Approve Redux?

At the time when Interneuron sought approval for Pondimin in the early 1970s, little was known about the link between fenfluramine and PPH. Only a few scattered case reports of PPH associated with fenfluramine surfaced in Europe, and they occurred after Pondimin was released in the United States. By the time Interneuron went back to the FDA to seek approval for Redux in 1994, however there was much more information regarding the PPH risk.[16,17,18]

Also during this period, Dr. Michael Weintraub had completed his landmark study of phen-fen. By 1995 enough doctors and patients knew about the idea to result in an explosion of phen-fen use. Clinics popped up all over the place, prescribing phen-fen to obese patients, with scant regard for the warnings about long-term use of phentermine and fenfluramine in the *Physicians' Desk Reference.* Experts at the FDA worried about unforeseen consequences of phen-fen. Dr. Weintraub's study involved only 121 patients, and physicians were on their way to prescribing phen-fen to millions of people on the basis of a single study on 121 patients! Never before in the history of medicine had so many people been given medicine by so many doctors on the basis of data on so few test subjects.

The FDA has a long tradition of opposing combination drug therapies. The fear had always been that drugs that are safe individually might interact in combination and produce dangerous side effects. Consequently, the FDA worried about phen-fen. Although it is time-consuming and expensive to test combination drug therapies, the public demand for speed in testing and approving new drug therapies has placed great pressure on the FDA to approve new therapies quickly and cheaply.

The FDA could do little to regulate the use of the phen-fen combination, because both medicines in the combination had been previously approved for use in the treatment of obesity. Doctors were within the law to prescribe them together. Physicians in the United States, by long-standing tradition, have been allowed to prescribe medicines outside of FDA-approved guidelines, with the understanding that they give up the umbrella of protection provided by those guidelines. The doctor's sacred responsibility is to the welfare of patients, and if that means prescribing medicines outside of FDA guidelines, most doctors, all the good ones, are willing to do it. Many medicines are, in fact, prescribed in this way, "off-indication." For instance, the medication known as Klonopin is often prescribed for anxiety, yet its only FDA-approved indication is for seizures. Tetracycline is used to treat rosacea, a nonbacterial skin disorder, when tetracycline is only FDA-approved as an antibiotic. Many other examples can be cited.

When Interneuron presented the FDA with the chance to approve Redux, a single-drug therapy for obesity that had been more thoroughly tested, the FDA was eager to approve it. FDA panel members were aware of the dangers of the increasing incidence of obesity in Americans. As good physicians they wanted to help, and they wanted to reassert the primacy of the FDA in defining safe use of medications in the obesity field.

What happened next is described in the September 23, 1996, issue of *Time* magazine:[19]

> Then Interneuron went after and got FDA approval, a ruling that critics charge was made with unseemly—and perhaps unprofessional—haste. Says Lewis Seiden, a University of Chicago pharmacologist who testified before the FDA advisory committee: "The procedures were loose, to be mild about it."
>
> What Seiden and others claim is that the FDA glossed over evidence that both Redux and the older drug fenfluramine cause significant brain damage in laboratory animals, from mice to baboons . . .
>
> This potential danger, when combined with the generally acknowledged risk of PPH, was enough to persuade the FDA advisory committee to reject Redux by a five-to-three vote on the question of safety when it first came up for consideration a year ago. But a few hours later, FDA official Dr. James Bilstad reopened the discussion after some committee members had left the meeting. Since there was no longer a quorum, a new meeting was called for two months later, in November.
>
> When that time came, however, the anti-Redux forces were missing. The meeting had been scheduled—all too conveniently, they suggest—to coincide with an international neurosciences conference in San Diego. And at the second meeting, Redux won approval by a one-vote margin.

That, along with the fact that Interneuron sent a high-profile member of its Board of Directors, Alexander Haig, to the November meeting in what was perceived as a high-pressure lobbying effort, led to charges that Redux was moved through improperly.

Not so fast, counters the FDA's Bilstad. Yes, he did reopen the issue after last September's "no" vote. But that, he says, is because it became clear that the vote to reject was invalid: at least one member had misunderstood the wording of the question on the table. "Obviously," says Bilstad, "we wanted a nonambiguous recommendation from the committee." Some members had left the meeting, though, and without a quorum he couldn't proceed. He considered polling the absentees by phone, but the FDA counsel advised against doing so.

Hence the November meeting. Bilstad acknowledges that the schedule conflicted with the San Diego neurosciences conference. But since Seiden and other Redux opponents had thoroughly aired their views in September and had no new findings, Bilstad decided to go ahead. Says he: "We weighed the idea of putting off the decision for several months, until those experts could be there. Since the committee had heard their presentation before and were given transcripts, we decided that we had the benefit of their comments on the issues. It was a judgment call . . ."

"Besides," says Bilstad, "dexfenfluramine has been available in Europe for ten years, with some ten million users. It is highly unlikely that there is anything significant in toxicity to the drug that hasn't been picked up with this kind of experience."

The advisory committee's recommendation wasn't legally binding on FDA commissioner David Kessler. Last

December, twenty-two neuroscientists, including Seiden and Dr. George Ricaurte of Johns Hopkins, asked the FDA to "forgo a final decision on dexfenfluramine until more information is available on its serotonin-neurotoxic potential in humans." Nevertheless, Kessler gave the go-ahead for Redux last spring.

If this story in *Time* is true, and if there is trouble with Redux-induced PPH in the future, FDA commissioners may have some explaining to do.

The FDA made its decision to approve Redux based on three assumptions:

1. Redux is more effective in treating obesity than previously available agents.
2. The frequency of PPH in the general population is one to four per million.
3. The use of Redux increases the chance of developing PPH only fivefold.

Evidence to support all three of these assumptions was tendered by the advocates of Redux. Yet less than a year after the FDA deliberations, new data have shown that all three assumptions were incorrect.

The Wyeth-Ayerst company was waiting in the wings to promote Redux. Wyeth had purchased A. H. Robins in 1989, acquiring with it the license for Pondimin. They were eager to get Redux, the "new" FDA-approved appetite suppressant, at a time when phen-fen had already opened the public's mind to the promise of drug therapy for obesity. An army of Wyeth "reps" went out to physicians' offices to promote Redux. There are still many physicians who have not heard of Dr. Weintraub and phen-fen, but there cannot be any left who have not heard of Redux! Wyeth did a superb job of getting Redux off the ground. They induced HMOs to put Redux on their lists of approved medicines and agree to pay for medical treatment of obesity. The drug is showing up on hospital pharmacy lists. To the extent that the Wyeth blitz loosened up regulatory knots impeding the use of appetite suppressants, the company has done the public a service.

The bottom line is that Redux may be effective in combating obesity, but it may cause PPH. Phen-fen is probably more effective than Redux for obesity, but the fenfluramine component in it may cause PPH and heart valve disease. At this time, we just don't know how severe the risk is.

Clearly there is a need for a weight-loss therapy that is both effective and free of PPH risk, and I believe phen-Prozac is the answer. Phen-Prozac is just as effective as phen-fen, more effective than Redux, and has no associated risk of PPH or heart valve disease. We'll look next at the components of phen-Prozac and how it was developed.

---

*Phen-Prozac is as effective as phen-fen, more effective than Redux, and phen-Prozac has no associated risk of PPH or heart valve disease.*

---

# Toby's Story

## PART 4

WHEN TOBY REACHED COLLEGE, she had piled 200 pounds onto her 5'4" frame. She had let herself go after her crash with Tim. She concentrated on her school work, accepting the friendship she received from girlfriends, but giving up on men. Her dorm room became a haven where lonely girls could console each other and discuss their homesickness and problems with men and school. Naturally, there was always plenty of junk food available to be shared among the girls at their gab sessions.

In her sophomore year, Toby found that her best friends were drifting off into the sororities or living with their boyfriends. She grew tired of the little clutch of misfits that gathered in her room. She pledged a sorority and tried to get back into the social scene. She began to take better care of her appearance. She still ate as she pleased, whenever she was hungry. The food in the dorms had been horrible—too starchy—and the campus was surrounded by fast food and pizza places. It was hard to find food anywhere that was healthful—not that she was particularly concerned with healthful eating. Food, healthful or not, was the only thing that brought her satisfaction and a temporary sense of well-being. In addition, Toby was still not doing any scheduled exercise, other than walking a lot on campus.

She attracted attention by cultivating a bellowing voice and outlandish behavior. She joined the drama club. She wore floppy hats, beads, and wild clothes. She told crude jokes, and a couple of times smoked a cigar at a party. She drank more than she should have. Toby had always had a pretty face and she attracted attention from several young men, but never for very long. They were in and out of her life quickly; she never permitted herself to get attached to any of them, expecting them to take off after a few nights together. They never disappointed her in that respect.

Toby never used any birth control and her periods were always irregular. There were many weeks when she worried whether she had gotten pregnant during one of her brief romantic encounters, but her period always came. She swore she would take some precautions. She didn't want to use birth control pills, fearing they would make her gain weight. Toby was afraid of getting pregnant in the future, even though she desperately wanted children someday. The weight she would gain from pregnancy made her apprehensive. She remembered her mother complaining about how fat she had gotten from her pregnancies. She had seen her mother's stretch marks and scar and did not want to have a C-section. The whole issue with men was fraught with danger and discomfort; sometimes she imagined that if there were no men in the world, the whole weight issue would go away. Women could relax and just be sisters.

Toby did not have much respect for men. None of them had ever appreciated her for what she was on the inside, only how she was shaped on the outside. At times she thought of using her weight to keep men away.

Her parents and friends had always told her that she was suffering from low self-esteem. They kept insisting on the fact, but she never believed it. Actually, Toby had quite high self-esteem. She knew she was intelligent and socially astute, even if the body in which her soul was packaged did not allow her to take full advantage of her talents. She had to work harder to get good grades from her male professors. She was turned down for summer jobs. Employers always made up excuses about why they didn't need her, but she was convinced of the real reason. She noticed it all—the world's cruel discrimination against overweight people—and it made her angry.

CHAPTER FIVE

# The Development of Phen-Prozac

Several years ago, before the idea of combining phentermine with Prozac entered my mind, I was introduced to phen-fen when some of my patients brought me copies of magazine articles touting its success. I was wary of the idea at first because I had had disappointing experiences with phentermine, which I had given by itself to about one hundred patients during the early years of my practice, with no lasting success. Patients lost a little weight at first, but gained it back even when they kept taking phentermine. At the time, I had no inkling that I could combine phentermine with Prozac to keep the weight loss going.

## How I Overcame My Resistance to Phentermine

Like many other physicians, I was originally discouraged from prescribing phentermine on a long-term basis by warnings in the *Physicians' Desk Reference (PDR)*.[1] The *PDR* is often called the "Doctor's Bible," though it is not as useful to doctors as people might think. Like the Bible, it is a large book written at different times by many different authors, and much of the data in the *PDR* is as old as Deuteronomy. The articles about each medicine are written by the pharmaceutical company that produces the medicine. You might expect the companies to give glowing reviews of their products, toning down risks to avoid scaring off consumers, but pharmaceutical companies are more worried about liability than losing customers. They issue warnings on every rare side effect, chance association, and theoretical concern they can think of. This practice makes the *PDR* of limited use to physicians.

On the subject of phentermine, for instance, the *PDR* says:

> Phentermine is indicated in the management of exogenous obesity as a short-term (a few weeks) adjunct in a regimen of weight reduction based on caloric restriction. The limited usefulness of agents of this class should be measured against possible risk factors inherent in their use such as those described below . . .
>
> . . . Tolerance to the anorectic effect usually develops within a few weeks. When this occurs, the recommended dose should not be exceeded in an attempt to increase the effect; rather, the drug should be discontinued . . .

. . . Drug Dependence: Phentermine is related chemically and pharmacologically to the amphetamines. Amphetamines and related stimulant drugs have been extensively abused, and the possibility of abuse should be kept in mind when evaluating the desirability of including a drug as part of a weight reduction program . . ."

These paragraphs are followed by a list of reputed ill effects of phentermine. All the serious side effects—addiction, dangerous arrhythmias of the heart, and others in the list—were derived from published studies of old addictive amphetamines, not direct studies of the new, safer medicine, phentermine itself.

The word *amphetamine* is the name of a large class of drugs that share the same chemical backbone. The name for the class "amphetamine" derives from the chemical name for this backbone: *Alpha-Methyl-beta-PHenyl-EThyl-AMINE.* The neurotransmitters dopamine and noradrenalin are examples of naturally occurring amphetamines. Popular over-the-counter nasal decongestants such as pseudoephedrine (Sudafed) and phenylpropanolamine (Dimetapp and Contac) are also amphetamines.

The parent drug of the amphetamine class is Dexedrine. Some other, old members of the class are Benzadrine and Methadrine. All three of these agents are powerful, addictive substances that were frequently abused in the sixties. Benzadrine tablets were called "Bennies" and Methadrine was called "Meth." Only Dexedrine is still used by physicians today, cautiously, in some patients with attention deficit disorder or narcolepsy.

Obviously, not all the amphetamines are addictive. No one is seriously worried about Sudafed and Contac, and dopamine and noradrenalin occur naturally in the brain. But the *PDR* claimed that "amphetamines and related stimulant drugs have been extensively abused, and the possibility of abuse should be kept in mind . . ." I heeded the sinister tone of that warning, assuming the authors of the *PDR* knew more about drugs than I did, and was thus inhibited from prescribing phentermine on a long-term basis to my obese patients.

The makers of phentermine may have protected themselves from liability suits by exaggerating their warnings, but in so doing they sold their product short, held up obesity research for years, prompted costly malpractice suits against good physicians, and kept a useful therapy out of the hands of the American people. The fault does not lie solely with the drug companies; the FDA advises companies on what warnings to print.

## Phentermine Is Not Addictive

Why is it that some amphetamines, such as Dexedrine, are addictive and others are not? It turns out that all addictive drugs are addictive for the same reason: they promote the effect of dopamine in the posterior limbic lobe of the brain, in an area of the limbic lobe called the *nucleus acumbens.* Drugs as diverse as caffeine, cocaine, alcohol, and nicotine all promote the effect of dopamine in the limbic lobe.[2] The limbic lobe of the brain is devoted to pleasure-pain issues. The reason why we seek sexual pleasure and the reason we love chocolate has a lot to do with what goes on in the limbic lobe. In psychological terms, the limbic lobe is the seat of our drives.

Some people are genetically cursed with low levels of limbic dopamine, others develop low levels later in life. Such people are predisposed to drug addiction, and these unfortunate people often must be monitored closely to keep from self-destructing. Judges, prosecutors, jailers, and Drug Enforcement Agency agents would have a lot less to do (and we would save a lot of tax dollars) if we could find a way to elevate the dopamine levels of the estimated 20 percent of the population with low limbic dopamine, without causing addiction.

It may sound like a dream, but the dream may be nearer than you think. In May 1997, bupropion, a nonaddictive, antidepressant drug that modulates dopamine in several parts of the brain, was approved for use in helping patients quit smoking. Patients who used bupropion were twice as likely to kick the habit as patients who went cold turkey or used a nicotine patch.[3]

---

*Phentermine is a very weak releaser of dopamine in the limbic lobe. It is not addictive at all.*

---

The relevance to phentermine is this: Dexedrine is a strong releaser of dopamine in the limbic lobe and is therefore addictive. Phentermine is a very weak releaser of dopamine in the limbic lobe.[4,5] It is not addictive at all. There is not a single study anywhere to show that phentermine is addictive. I have not seen a single example of addiction with normal doses of phentermine; neither have Drs. Weintraub, Eig, Mirkin, Steelman, or Atkinson, and we have had ten thousand patients among us using phentermine.

Many of my patients on phen-Prozac found it easier to stop smoking or drinking. I didn't expect this—I didn't know about limbic dopamine back in 1995—but so many patients reported that they had gained control of their addictive habits that I am convinced it is a real effect. Several studies show that when rats were treated with phentermine before exposure to cocaine, they could be given cocaine without becoming addicted![6] Far from being addictive itself, phentermine may be a useful preventive treatment for addiction.[7,8]

The concept that all amphetamines are by nature addictive is obsolete. The amphetamine class of compounds now includes a wide range, many of which look nothing like the parent compound, Dexedrine. Some of these compounds are addictive, but most are not. Some release dopamine, but many do not. Some release serotonin, but others do not. The whole area is badly in need of a new classification scheme. It would be best if the term *amphetamine* was forgotten altogether. It has outlived its usefulness. Recognizing this, the Drug Enforcement Agency has transferred phentermine from Schedule III (addictive drugs) to Schedule IV (non-addicting drugs).

## Phentermine Needs a Partner

Phentermine has been on the market for thirty years, but it had negligible impact on obesity until it was teamed with fenfluramine. Phentermine given alone suppresses the appetite for a few weeks, but the excess appetite always returns, and the lost weight is regained. The important, central lesson of Dr. Weintraub's work was that when phentermine was combined with fenfluramine, which is a serotonin-promoting drug, the appetite suppressant effect of phentermine was significantly prolonged.

*Phentermine has been on the market for thirty years, but it had negligible impact on obesity until it was teamed with fenfluramine.*

Serotonin is another naturally occurring neurotransmitter in the brain. Serotonin is involved in the brain centers associated with sleep, feelings of well-being, sex drive, and appetite. Everyone in America experiences the effects of serotonin after a Thanksgiving turkey dinner. They feel sleepy, happy, unsexy, and well-fed, all the result of an increase in brain serotonin caused by eating turkey. Turkey meat protein contains a high proportion of tryptophan, the starting material for serotonin synthesis. Eating turkey and other high-tryptophan foods increases brain serotonin. Judith Wurtman, Ph.D., wrote a book, *The Serotonin Solution* (Fawcett Columbine, New York, 1996), proposing that obese people could feel full before they had actually overeaten by sticking to high-tryptophan foods. This approach is not practical because most high-tryptophan foods, prepared the way ordinary people like them, are high in fat and calories. Nevertheless, the idea serves as a nice introduction to serotonin.

Dr. Weintraub did not choose fenfluramine to use with phentermine because of its serotonin-raising effect. He chose it only because it worked by a different mechanism from phentermine and it was FDA-approved for the treatment of obesity.

But it was serendipitous that he chose a serotonin-raising medicine to use with phentermine, because that was the key that made the whole thing work. If he had chosen diethylpropion (Tenuate) to use with phentermine, history would have been different.

There are a few other minor appetite suppressants in the United States that increase serotonin effect, such as phendimetrazine (Bontril). There are even more serotonin-active appetite suppressants in Europe.

Not all the medicines that increase serotonin are appetite suppressants. The old antidepresssants, such as amitryptiline (Elavil) and nortryptiline (Pamelor), increase serotonin in parts of the brain involved in depression. Their effect on the appetite center, however, is to increase appetite.

But there is a class of serotonin-active antidepressants that does not increase appetite. This class is the SSRIs (Selective Serotonin Reuptake Inhibitors). These were the medicines I focused on to find a partner for phentermine that would be safer and better than fenfluramine.

The SSRI drugs, of which Prozac is the most prominent member, were originally developed as antidepressants. They are now used to treat a variety of conditions, not only depression, because serotonin is involved in so many different functions of the brain. SSRI drugs are used to treat ADD (attention deficit disorder), autism, bulimia, PMS (premenstrual syndrome), migraine, insomnia, irritable bowel syndrome, premature ejaculation, and obsessive-compulsive disorder (OCD).

The use of SSRIs to treat obsessive-compulsive disorder caused me to consider an SSRI as a substitute for fenfluramine in the phen-fen program. I reasoned that an obese patient's obsession with food might be a form of obsessive-compulsive disorder. If Prozac was useful in treating OCD, why not obesity?

To understand what SSRIs do, you must learn a little biochemistry; it's worth the effort because neurotransmitters are more and more in the news. Just as you had to learn something about DNA to follow the O. J. Simpson trial, you'll have to know something about brain chemistry to keep up with the news. The chemical structure of Prozac reminded me of serotonin and fenfluramine, suggesting that Prozac might be an adequate substitute for fenfluramine. Here is what serotonin looks like to a chemist:

**Serotonin**

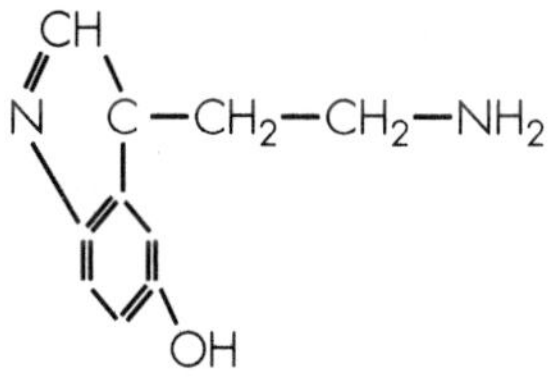


FIGURE 5.1

"C" stands for carbon, "N" for nitrogen, "O" for oxygen, and "H" for hydrogen, but don't worry about that. The thing to notice is the shape of the molecule, especially its right-hand side and the little hexagon underneath.

Now look at Prozac:

**Prozac**

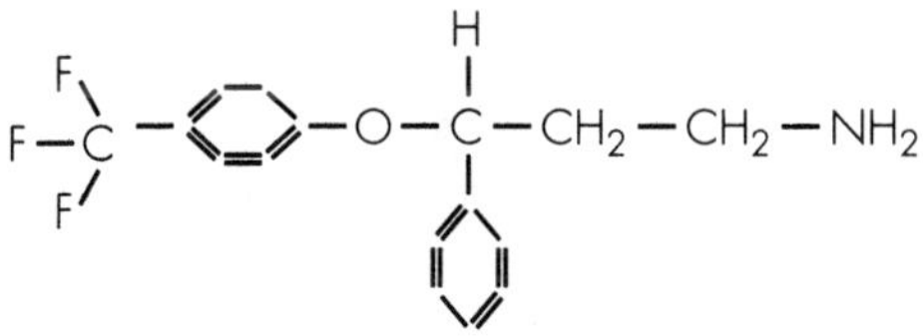


FIGURE 5.2

The chemical structure of Prozac is very similar to that of serotonin. In fact, the right-hand side of the Prozac molecule is identical to that of serotonin. "F" stands for fluorine.

What does serotonin do in the brain? It is a chemical messenger that transmits nerve impulses across the spaces between nerve cells, called synapses. After serotonin has done its job in the synapse, it is pumped back into the nerve cell by a special "serotonin pump" on the surface of the presynaptic nerve cell.

As you may know, the predominant theory about the cause of depression is that the brains of individuals with depression are low in serotonin, impairing the transmission of nerve impulses. Prozac promotes the effect of serotonin by blocking the membrane pump that pumps serotonin back into the presynaptic nerve cell. More serotonin is left in the synapse longer, guaranteeing better transmission of nerve impulses. The diagram in Figure 5.3 makes this clear:

**The Action of SSRI Medicines on Nerve Cell Connections in the Brain**

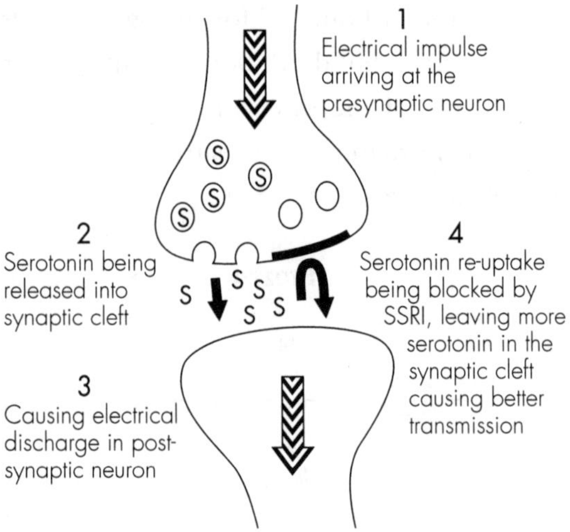
1
Electrical impulse arriving at the presynaptic neuron
2
Serotonin being released into synaptic cleft
3
Causing electrical discharge in post-synaptic neuron
4
Serotonin re-uptake being blocked by SSRI, leaving more serotonin in the synaptic cleft causing better transmission
S

FIGURE 5.3

Fenfluramine has similarities with Prozac, and some important differences.

**Fenfluramine, Redux, Pondimin**

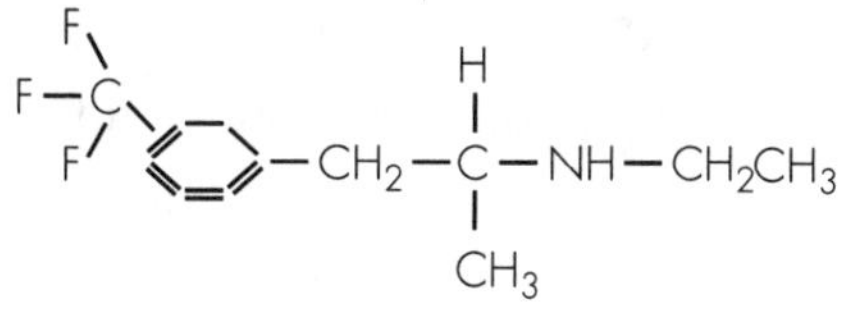

FIGURE 5.4

Fenfluramine is not an SSRI. Instead, it rides into the presynaptic nerve cell through the same pump affected by Prozac, without blocking the pump. Once inside, fenfluramine causes direct release of a burst of serotonin into the synapse. This makes fenfluramine a very potent serotonin-promoting drug, but it also produces more side effects and enables it to cause PPH. Remember, as we discussed in Chapter 4, Prozac does not cause PPH.

## Phen-Prozac Breakthrough

I did not know about fenfluramine-induced PPH in March of 1995, when I was contemplating magazine articles my patients brought me regarding phen-fen and Dr. Weintraub. I was worried that fenfluramine might cause the patients unacceptable diarrhea and cost too much money. Many patients had prescription cards that would not cover fenfluramine because HMO insurance companies, in their frugal wisdom, defined obesity as a "cosmetic problem" to avoid paying for its care. Phentermine was not a problem—it was cheap—but fenfluramine could cost as much as $60 a month.

Then it struck me: why use fenfluramine at all? Prozac had all the advantages. Fenfluramine has a shorter half-life than Prozac; it doesn't stay in the body as long, so fenfluramine has to be dosed two or three times a day. Prozac needs to be taken only once a day and generally has less side effects than fenfluramine. Prescription cards often did not cover fenfluramine, but all covered Prozac. For patients who could not afford Prozac (at $2.50 per 10-mg pill), the Eli Lilly company was generous in supplying samples, which I could dispense at my discretion to defray the expense. Obese patients with depression could have the obesity and depression treated at the same time. Fenfluramine is not an effective antidepressant.

I started prescribing phen-Prozac to obese patients in March 1995. I randomly assigned half my patients to phen-fen and half to phen-Prozac, to see which program worked best.

---

*For weight loss, only 10 mg of Prozac per day are needed.*

---

While higher doses of Prozac are needed to treat depression, the lowest dose of Prozac suffices to generate the maximum weight loss in patients taking phen-Prozac. Typical doses of Prozac for depressed patients are 20 to 40 mg per day. Obsessive-compulsive disorder patients get 40 to 80 mg per day. For weight loss, only 10 mg per day are needed. This more than anything else has convinced me that Prozac does not produce weight loss by curing depression, or OCD coexisting with depression, but by a direct effect on the appestat. This pleasant fact meant that my patients almost never experienced side effects from Prozac. The few side effects encountered were from the phentermine.

By August, I had given the medicines to sixty patients, and I was impressed by the results. Most patients lost one to two pounds per week, steadily. Phen-Prozac and phen-fen worked equally well in generating weight loss, but the patients taking phen-Prozac experienced fewer side effects and spent less money.

At that point I made two decisions. First, to prescribe only phen-Prozac for my patients. Second, to contact obese patients in my practice to inform them about the program. If it was good for some, it should be offered to all. There was no reason to withhold it from any obese patient for whom there was no contraindication to the therapy.

By November of 1995, I had treated two hundred people with phen-Prozac. The first set of phen-Prozac patients were reaching ideal body weight and staying there. Twenty-five percent required no more medication to keep their weight low. The rest needed a small dose of phen-Prozac to stay at the new reduced weight. Enthusiasm was high. Patients seldom missed a dose.

## Does This Program Work with Other SSRIs?

Prozac was not the only SSRI drug I prescribed. Some of my obese patients who were already taking an antidepressant to treat depression asked if they had to stop their old antidepressant to go on Prozac. Since most of their antidepressants were SSRIs, like Prozac, I reasoned that their old antidepressant might work as well as Prozac for weight loss. My supposition proved correct. At this time, I have a large number of patients taking phentermine combined with Zoloft, trazodone, Luvox, and many other SSRIs, all experiencing success. Access to alternative SSRIs also gave me greater ability to eliminate SSRI-related side effects by substituting one SSRI for another. Physicians who prescribe only fenfluramine do not have this flexibility.

Not all SSRIs have worked in my experience thus far. The old tricyclic antidepressants, such as Elavil and Pamelor, did

*I have a large number of patients taking phentermine combined with Zoloft, trazodone, Luvox, and many other SSRIs, all experiencing success.*

not work because they themselves stimulated appetite. Paxil was also a flop; there was no weight loss even though it is a first cousin to Prozac and Zoloft. Wellbutrin did not work either. But these conclusions are preliminary. I have far more experience with phen-Prozac than with the other combinations.

## Getting the Word Out

Convinced of its effectiveness, I discussed phen-Prozac with fellow physicians. I called Dr. Weintraub and invited him to speak to physicians at a Thursday lunch conference at my local hospital. He accepted, but the talk was delayed several times. (First Newt Gingrich kindly shut down the federal government and sent Dr. Weintraub and the rest of the FDA on furlough. Then the lecture was held up by the infamous blizzard of '96.)

Meanwhile, I started to accept obese patients from other doctors who were unwilling to prescribe combination appetite suppressant therapy themselves. Phen-fen was becoming so well known to the public that patients were breaking down the doors of physicians willing to prescribe the program. Phen-fen weight-loss clinics opened and advertised in newspapers and magazines. The Rader Institute in California sought to enroll physicians in all fifty states to administer phen-fen in their Comprehensive Weight Control Clinics (CWCC). Even Jenny Craig and Nutrasystems, after years of resistance to medical therapy, jumped on the bandwagon, contracting with physicians to prescribe phen-fen to clients.

By spring of 1996, I was surprised that most of my fellow mainstream physicians were still blithely unaware of phen-anything, and even displayed intolerance for the concept of medical therapy for obesity, which I advocated at medical meetings. It was as though I were proposing religious heresy. Would they have been so emotional if I were proposing an alternative therapy for diabetes or gout?[9] But I was striking a raw nerve, a deep-running current that said that overweight people were fat because they deserved to be. Obesity was their "just reward" for being such "bad" patients. Offering them an easy way out was immoral—one doctor actually said that to me! I was offering patients a "magic pill," he declared, and felt sure that it would disappoint them in the end. If you think that attitude is sick, so do I!

Dr. Weintraub delivered his long-awaited lecture at Shady Grove Hospital in April of 1996, and the assembly of physicians was impressed. After that, I delivered lectures at three local hospitals. I published an article in *Archives of Internal Medicine* describing my results.[10]

No doctor in my part of Maryland can have failed to hear about phen-Prozac by now. I have treated 548 patients with a high rate of success and perfect safety. Spreading the word to the rest of America remains: obese people need no longer be steered away from medical therapy.

## FDA Approval

Combination appetite suppressants have strong advantages over single agents. I encouraged the Eli Lilly company, manufacturer of Prozac, to seek FDA approval for the phen-Prozac combination for obesity therapy, but after conferring with high-level officials at the company, I am sorry to report that the company will never do so. The patent for Prozac will expire in the year 2002, and officials at Eli Lilly know they won't make much money from Prozac once the patent expires and competing companies produce generic versions. To get FDA approval for the phen-Prozac combination, the company would have to present studies showing the efficacy as well as the safety of the combination, even though Prozac and phentermine are known to be safe separately.

Furthermore, the officials informed me that Eli Lilly has other drugs in the pipeline that may be as effective as phen-Prozac, with shiny new patents, which promise to generate profits for a longer period of time.

I carried my case to the Pfizer company of Philadelphia, makers of Zoloft, but encountered the same problem there. Not enough time. Not enough profit.

It might help if I explain what FDA approval does and doesn't mean. Companies need FDA approval for specific indications (uses of the drug) before they can advertise it for those indications. Approval from the FDA is not blanket approval for all purposes. Prozac, for instance, is indicated for depression and OCD only. In advertising, Eli Lilly can claim only that Prozac is effective in treating depression and OCD. Prozac is known to relieve symptoms of PMS and doctors may prescribe Prozac for PMS, but Eli Lilly, in its advertising, cannot claim that Prozac works in treating PMS.

Eli Lilly will make its $3.25 for each 20-mg Prozac capsule sold, whether it is prescribed for depression or PMS. The patient who uses Prozac for PMS will experience the benefit. So what's the problem?

The problem is that institutional prescribers, such as Jenny Craig, Kaiser Permanente, or Medicare/Medicaid, are restricted to prescribing medicines according to FDA guidelines. Doctors who prescribe outside these guidelines are at legal risk. FDA guidelines would work better if the actual medical potential of drugs was held in higher esteem than the economic concerns of the manufacturer. Why should the fact that the patent for Prozac expires in the year 2002 have anything to do with FDA approval of phen-Prozac for weight loss therapy?

### A Nation of Barbies and Kens?

Phen-Prozac can help nearly all obese Americans reach their safe weight range, that is, a BMI lower than 25. But should we go a step farther and insist on reducing to the point that everyone of the same height wears the same size? Should we try to become a nation of Barbies and Kens? That is not the goal, for the following reasons.

1. Economics. While the savings in health care and productivity from getting all obese patients into a safe weight range would be enormous, there would be no economic benefit from getting people already in the BMI 19–25 range down to their dream dress or pants size. Prozac costs $3+ per pill. With health costs rising steeply and many people denied basic health care, it seems poor economy to waste health dollars on cosmetic weight adjustments.

2. Medical prudence. Phen-fen and phen-Prozac are relatively new therapies. The component medicines have been well tested, but the combination is new. Although we can safely say that the known risks of phen-fen, phen-Prozac, or Redux do not outweigh the known risks of severe obesity, at this early stage, we cannot be sure that the risk/benefit ratio is sufficiently favorable for those seeking a strictly cosmetic reduction in weight.

3. Jurisprudence. No doctor should treat people who are mildly obese with Redux or phen-anything, because if there is

---

*Should we insist that everyone of the same height wears the same size? Should we try to become a nation of Barbies and Kens?*

---

an adverse event—even one not related to the therapy—the doctor may be exposed to a malpractice suit. State medical boards are in turmoil over the use of appetite suppressants. Before extending drug therapy to mildly obese individuals, let's be sure it is medically and legally warranted.

4. Biological reality. Use of phen-Prozac does not in every case achieve the desired weight or dress size. Phen-fen and phen-Prozac seem to work only on the abnormal component of appetite, so the therapy can get everyone into the BMI 19–25 range, but it can't make every woman a size 4.

5. Philosophical objection. Do we honestly want everyone to have the same body size? Diversity is good, as long as it is healthy diversity. Negative futuristic depictions of the human race in movies like *1984* and *Brazil* show human beings reduced to uniform shapes and colors, everyone wearing gray suits and dull expressions. I hope to never see such a situation. May we always have variety in our character and our looks: blondes and brunettes, dark skin and light, thin and heavy—just not heavy to the point of being unhealthy.

# Toby's Story

## PART 5

Toby thought she had lost a little weight in her senior year of college, but the scale still read 240 pounds when she graduated. She intended to go to business school, but decided to go to work in a bank to gain practical experience. She knew she had a good head for business, but worried that she might have trouble finding a job after business school; none of the women she saw in business magazines or interviews were her size. There must have been a reason for that.

But Toby would not have been satisfied with letting her weight get in the way of her ambition indefinitely. She told herself that the job at the bank was temporary work to gain experience and to earn extra money to support herself in business school later. However, she couldn't help feeling disappointed by her decision.

The fact of her obesity pressed in on her. She was sick of having nothing to wear. Her closet was full of clothes of varying sizes from her "thinner days"—she would wear them when she lost weight. She was tired of underwear that looked like sails, brassieres that looked like parachutes. Tired of sweating. Tired of having to shop in the "plus size" section of the department store. Her bedroom slippers were crushed flat as tortillas, and she could never find a comfortable pair of shoes for her aching feet. She went everywhere in tennis shoes or flip-flops.

It was at this point that she consulted a physician for the first time about her weight. Dr. Cab was an internist. Like most internists, he had had no training in nutrition, diet, or exercise in medical school or residency, but Toby didn't know that. She assumed that these were very important subjects in medical school, since obesity is related to so many diseases.

Dr. Cab tried to tell her at first that all she needed to do was to eat "lite" and get some exercise. Toby did not let him get off so easily. She assured him that she had already tried low-fat diets and exercise, and they had not worked. This was not strictly true. She had not remained on diets very long because she had become very hungry. She felt fairly certain that medical science with all its touted technology would have something more sophisticated to help her.

Dr. Cab prescribed the Optifast System for her. This was a system of liquid meals, similar to the Nutrasystem diet, but prescribed through the offices of private physicians. Dr. Cab directed Toby to drink the liquid supplement at breakfast and lunch, but to eat a regular supper. He didn't want her to get all of her nutrition from the liquid supplements, because in the past there had been fatalities from total diets of high-protein liquid substances. What Dr. Cab did not know was that Toby had always eaten almost all her calories at night. So the liquid supplement, instead of replacing one or two meals, was actually added on to Toby's customary caloric intake; the drink seemed to have little effect on her nighttime hunger. Not surprisingly then, it failed.

Toby's exercise program was a failure, too. She had taken up walking around her block in the mornings. She had good shoes, but the only surface to walk on was the sidewalk, and she developed tendonitis of the feet and sore knees. That put an end to the walking program. It was physically difficult to ride a bicycle and swimming didn't provide much exercise.

After a few months of the diet program, her weight was pushing 260. Dr. Cab was not happy to see her back. (In fact, in several polls in which physicians were asked which category of patient was their least favorite to see, obese patients scored first or second.) Dr. Cab was typical of physicians in that respect, but he also felt he had a duty to his patient. She would not listen to any more advice about diet and exercise, so he prescribed Ionamin, a brandname form of phentermine 30 mg. The prescription was very expensive. Toby made the mistake of starting the therapy on a Monday. Insomnia was one of the side effects of the medication for some people, and she couldn't sleep all week. By Thursday she was too exhausted to go to work.

The Ionamin certainly eliminated her appetite, and she was willing to put up with the side effects for that. She was desperate. The side effects abated and she had two great weeks during which she lost ten pounds. The third week, however, she lost only two pounds. The fourth week she lost one pound. The fifth week she gained two pounds. In fact, she lost no more weight even though she continued to take the Ionamin. The Ionamin was very expensive, and when it came time to refill it she had second thoughts. She was not losing any more weight, and Dr. Cab was unwilling to keep prescribing it. He said it was addictive; not good for the long term. As a matter of fact, Dr. Cab didn't seem very interested in her problem at all anymore.

CHAPTER SIX

# A Closer Look at Phentermine and Prozac

Now that you have a grasp of the significance of phen-Prozac in weight-loss treatment, let's look more closely at the nature of its components and how this program might work for you.

## Good and Bad Side Effects of Phentermine

Phentermine is not addictive, but it does cause mild, reversible side effects in some people. The most common side effects are those you might expect from a stimulant medication, even caffeine or Sudafed.

Phentermine can cause nervousness, fast heartbeat, and insomnia. These side effects frequently occur when phentermine is started abruptly at a dose of 30 mg or more. I have learned to always start phentermine at a lower dose (15 mg) for one or two weeks before progressing to the usual effective dose of 30 mg. In this way, the stimulant side effects of phentermine are reduced or avoided. Do not assume that your physician will know this. If your physician prescribes phentermine for you, ask about using half-dose pills to begin the therapy.

Phentermine can cause constipation. SSRI drugs have the opposite effect: they tend to cause diarrhea. The constipation-tendency of phentermine is offset by the diarrhea-tendency of the SSRI, and the result is regular bowel movements. Other typical side effects of phentermine are offset by the SSRI in the same way. In fact, the combination of phentermine and an SSRI has been consistently better tolerated than either medicine alone.

Phentermine can cause a dry mouth. Patients taking phentermine deal with the dryness problem by drinking more water—but that's good news! Most American adults don't drink enough water. Children and teenagers take time off to gulp down a glass of water at the sink, but adults seldom do. They insist instead on coffee, tea, or other beverages that cost money and come in little cups. And the little paper cones by the office water cooler are ridiculous! We are a dehydrated nation. We pee yellow. And we pay for it with kidney stones in men and urinary tract infections in women. Patients who are losing weight need to drink more water than usual, because they are using water to break down fat. Forty-eight molecules of water are required to hydrolyze each molecule of triolein, the most common component of body fat.

Phentermine dries up the nasal passages, and this is usually a good side effect too. Many of my obese patients with chronic allergies, sinusitis, or vasomotor rhinitis have reported to me that they could breathe more easily on phentermine. In fact, patients who take phentermine should not take nasal decongestants such as Sudafed or Contac for a cold, because the decongestants in those products are also stimulants. Taking them together with phentermine can cause additive side effects. Patients prone to nosebleeds in the winter should keep their nasal passages moist with nasal saline while taking phentermine. Nasal saline drops are available over the counter.

Both nasal decongestants and phentermine can cause swelling of the prostate gland. Men with enlarged prostates should consult a urologist before taking phentermine.

Phentermine can cause increased sweating. My patients seldom complain of sweating, however, because they are accustomed to the fat around their middle acting like an overcoat. Over time, after losing weight with phen-Prozac, most patients will notice a reduction in the sweating. For patients whose excess sweating is confined to a particular part of the body, some effective remedies are described later in this book, in the table of side effects in Chapter 12.

The *PDR* claims that phentermine can cause euphoria and rare psychotic disturbances, but those statements are borrowed from studies of more potent amphetamines such as Dexedrine. I have never observed these side effects in my patients, and no doctor I have talked with has witnessed them either.

## Observations on Side Effects

I am continually amazed by how many patients won't take life-saving prescription medications because they are afraid of side effects. Yet many of these same people will flock to health food stores to purchase untested folk remedies or spend fortunes on vitamin supplements and minerals. I only wish as many obese people would take phen-Prozac as take garlic, melatonin, and chromium picolinate.

There are two types of side effects. The most common are the reversible side effects. These are side effects that clear up completely once the medication is stopped. Phentermine has several reversible side effects, such as insomnia or nausea, nothing too serious when weighed against the benefits. The less common type are the irreversible side effects, which do not go away when the medication is stopped. Phentermine has no known side effects of this type.

*Phentermine has no known irreversible side effects.*

Side effects will not occur in all people who take a particular medicine. This might seem obvious, but many people expect that they will automatically experience every side effect ever reported for a drug, when this is rarely the case. Any medicine that creates significant side effects in all users would never make it to market in the first place. The FDA system of drug approval works well in that respect.

## Concerns About Prozac

It seems to me that more people in this country remember the Prozac Scare than Operation Desert Storm, both of which occurred in 1991. The Prozac Scare, to this day, makes it difficult to convince patients that a Prozac prescription can be safe.

Prozac appeared on the U.S. market in 1987 and rose to a preeminent place among antidepressants because of its efficacy, speed of onset, and low side-effect profile. The future for Eli Lilly's product seemed rosy back then.

But it wasn't long before a report of six cases of suicidal behavior in patients taking Prozac surfaced in the *American Journal of Psychiatry*.[1] In response to that report, physicians and scientists began a methodical investigation. A series of editorials appeared in the *American Journal of Psychiatry*, followed by several large statistical studies of Prozac and other antidepressants—which exonerated Prozac.[2]

The process of follow-up and study is ongoing, but the majority opinion at present seems to be that Prozac and some other serotonin-active antidepressants may initially depress brain serotonin, which can make the depression temporarily worse in certain depressed patients. There is no evidence, and there has never been a scientific claim, that Prozac incited suicidal behavior in patients who were not depressed to begin with. That's such an important statement that I think I'll say it again: there has never been a claim that Prozac incited suicidal behavior in patients who were not depressed to begin with.

Physicians have circumvented the problem of initial depression of serotonin in some patients by starting antidepressant therapy with Prozac at a low dose of 10 mg for the first few weeks before progressing to the usual antidepressant dose of 20 mg. This is a safe procedure in patients with both obesity and depression, for whom Prozac is doing double duty. Obese patients without depression are not given a dose of Prozac higher than 10 mg anyway. Scientists and doctors have a way of working out problems based on data and reason that can prevail in a peaceful atmosphere away from the spotlight of public attention.

Unfortunately, in 1991 the Church of Scientology placed a series of advertisements in *USA Today* claiming that Prozac caused suicides, homicides, and domestic violence. National news media picked up the story, paying scant attention to its source—after all, they say negative stories get better ratings than positive ones. Oprah Winfrey hosted Peter Breggin, author of *Talking Back to Prozac,* and Phil Donahue presented an eager Prozac doomsayer on his show.

The Church of Scientology, encouraged by the response to its advertising campaign, acting through a subgroup, the Citizens Commission on Human Rights, petitioned the FDA to cancel approval of Prozac. The FDA looked over the data carefully and saw no reason to withdraw its support for Prozac.[3]

The whole story was told in articles in *Time*[4] and *The Wall Street Journal,*[5,6,7] but refutations of the charges were not broadcast as prominently as the original charges. Eli Lilly lost millions of dollars in sales, and thousands of patients went off their antidepressant medication, suffering terribly as a result. Many suicides and homicides resulted from *not* taking Prozac. To complete the fiasco, many violent criminals who had taken Prozac claimed in their defense that it was Prozac that made them commit those crimes.[8] It is a tribute to the American system of justice that not one of these defendants prevailed in court.

Nearly half of all patients in the U.S. who take an antidepressant take Prozac. After ten years of use, mainstream physicians have been convinced by its results to have full confidence in the medicine. If the problems alleged by Scientologists held any validity, they would have been proven by now. Physicians would have no reason to hide the problems of Prozac; all they want is to make their patients well and get home by 8 o'clock. I know it's true. I'm a physician myself.

*After ten years of use, mainstream physicians have been convinced by its results to have full confidence in Prozac.*

### The American View of Mental Illness

Aside from the Prozac Scare, a more general problem is apparent in the way Americans view mental illness and the medicines used to treat it. Many obese patients are hesitant to go on phen-Prozac because they fear, with good reason, that if their insurance carrier finds out they are taking an "antidepressant," their insurance premiums will be raised. Under Federal Aviation Administration (FAA) rules, pilots who test positive for Prozac are grounded.[9] Now, who would you prefer to have in the cockpit: a pilot whose depression has been successfully treated by a physician, or a pilot who is afraid to admit to being depressed? Depression affects 20 percent of the population, so it probably affects about 20 percent of pilots. Wishing it weren't so does not make the problem go away.

Too many people, who don't know better, think that all mental illnesses are severe and debilitating. That isn't so. There are degrees of depression, just as there are degrees of influenza. To ground all pilots with a diagnosis of mental illness or to raise the insurance rates of every person with a diagnosis of depression, without considering the severity of the disease, is foolish. We know so much more about mental illness now than we did in 1900; it's time our policies reflected that knowledge.

## Beginnings of a Shift in Consciousness

This book and others teach that obesity, once thought to be under voluntary control, is not under voluntary control at all. Obese patients have no more control of their body weight than they have of their blood pressure. Yet no one blames patients with high blood pressure for their disease; no company raises their insurance premium if their blood pressure is well controlled, and the FAA doesn't suspend their pilot's license.

Individuals, companies, and regulatory agencies must recognize that this wonderful class of medicines—the SSRIs—has many uses beyond the treatment of depression. One should not assume that a person is unstable simply because he or she is taking Prozac. The person may not suffer from depression at all; Prozac is being used to effectively treat other conditions that have nothing to do with mental illness.

## Additional Benefits of Phen-Prozac

Not only can phentermine and Prozac be the core of effective, healthful weight-loss therapy, these medications have been found to affect a number of other conditions positively as well.

## Phentermine and ADD

Phentermine is an effective treatment for attention deficit disorder (ADD). ADD is a common biochemical brain disorder that causes patients to have difficulty concentrating on work and to have poor control of impulses. If the patient is hyperactive as well, the condition is called attention deficit hyperactivity disorder (ADHD).

Most people are familiar with this disorder in children. At lunchtime in almost every school, there is a line of boys and girls outside the school nurse's door, waiting to receive their midday dose of Ritalin, the most common medicine used to treat ADD. By the time boys reach sixth grade, half of them have been referred by their teachers for evaluation for ADD. ADD has been called the disease of the decade, but only 10 percent of boys and 1 percent of girls actually have the chemical component of the disorder.

Most children with ADD grow up to be adults with ADD. Because so many children have it, common sense would tell you that a lot of adults do, too. But few adults recognize the disorder in themselves or seek treatment for it. Adults with ADD are usually chronic underachievers in life. Many have difficulty with reading and writing because ADD made it difficult for them to learn these skills properly in school. They seek jobs where reading skills are less important; such jobs often pay poorly. Their marriages are destabilized by their hyperactivity and inattention.

Some of my patients taking phen-Prozac reported that they could concentrate on their work and control their impulses better. Many of these patients were living with unrecognized ADD, revealed by the improvement in its symptoms while taking phentermine. When I substituted phentermine for

Ritalin in obese young people with established ADD, phentermine worked as well for the ADD symptoms, and the patients lost weight. I was not the first to discover that phentermine treats ADD. The connection had been previously published.[10]

---

*Some patients taking phen-Prozac reported that they could concentrate on their work and control their impulses better.*

---

Of all the patients in my practice, those with adult ADD have been the most grateful because, serendipitously, the medication enabled them to get control of impulsive behaviors that had been out of control, while helping to reduce their obesity.

### SSRIs and Obsessive-Compulsive Disorder

My obese patients who also have obsessive-compulsive disorder reported substantial improvement in the OCD symptoms when they started the phen-Prozac program. Patients who have OCD cannot control their thoughts and impulses. "Obsessions" are thoughts the patient feels compelled to think. "Compulsions" are repeated ritual acts the patient feels compelled to perform. Most people have heard about the little boy who couldn't stop washing his hands or the night watchman who couldn't go home because he had to keep checking the doors in his building.

OCD is not the same disease as depression, although many patients with depression demonstrate elements of OCD. Many "normal" people have elements of OCD as well. We all have occasional obsessive thoughts or compulsions.

The current preferred medicine for treating OCD is Prozac. Luvox, a newcomer in the U.S. market, has also been approved for use in treating OCD. Other SSRIs probably work just as well. Most psychiatrists say that the dose of SSRI required to treat OCD is higher than that required to treat depression or obesity, but that may not be so. It may just be that patients seen by psychiatrists are afflicted with a higher degree of the disease. Patients who have the most common symptoms of OCD seldom go to the doctor to complain of their thoughts and actions. It is more characteristic of the disease that its sufferers have little insight into it. All they want is to go on thinking their obsessive thoughts and performing their compulsive acts; they are afraid that the doctor will try to make them stop.

Individuals with mild or moderate OCD have been enormously helped by the small doses of SSRI used to treat obesity. One patient taking phen-Prozac confessed to me, in mid-therapy, that she'd had a compulsion to buy compact discs. She had purchased ten thousand CDs! Neither she nor her husband had told me about this compulsive behavior, until she started taking phen-Prozac for obesity and unexpectedly gained control of the compulsion, as a side effect. She sold the CDs to a local radio station and ended up losing ninety-four pounds on the weight-loss program.

Some phen-Prozac patients report that they have mastered the compulsion to shop or to use credit cards excessively.

Others report less brooding, better control of their thoughts, and less anger.

OCD may have nothing to do with drug, alcohol, or tobacco addiction, but it is clear that patients who are taking phen-Prozac have an easier time quitting these harmful habits. There are ongoing studies of the use of phentermine, fenfluramine, and Prozac, alone and in various combinations, in treating addictions of all types,[11,12] and it will be interesting to see if this develops into a genuine solution to the serious problems caused by addictions.

# Toby's Story

## PART 6

AT SOME POINT, Toby became less interested in her weight problem. She was more interested, instead, in Frank Perrino, a young man with his own computer business who dropped in at the bank every day to make a deposit. Frank always waited to talk to Toby.

Toby noticed that Frank was on the overweight side, too. Or rather she didn't notice. She made a point of not noticing, because he was so nice to her. Her apartment was lonely. She was tired of watching television and feeling isolated.

Frank and Toby were married a year later. Toby had tried to lose weight to get into her wedding dress. By going hungry and walking every day at noon, she had made it; but the efforts were short lived because she got pregnant shortly after her wedding. She had been worried whether she was fertile. During college she might have gotten pregnant several times but never had. But Frank, it seemed, had her number. She was relieved in a way, but her old fears of pregnancy returned as she watched the numbers climb on the bathroom scale.

There is not much to say about Toby and Frank's first year together. They loved each other and had fun together, but their overweight condition was a constant burden to both of them. Frank hurt his back trying to carry Toby across the threshold. Toby sprained her ankle at the hotel during their honeymoon and got a urinary tract infection that took two courses of antibiotics to cure. She worried that she might have diabetes.

It was evident from the first few months of marriage that Frank was a workaholic. He spent most of his time at the office, massaging his business to produce more money for his family. Toby got home from work early, but not knowing when Frank was going to arrive, she didn't prepare meals. She got into baking breads and desserts instead. She suspected Frank ate at fast food restaurants, but she didn't ask.

She went regularly to the obstetrician, who kept careful tabs on her weight. He explained to her that the pregnancy was at increased risk because of her weight. In spite of all her efforts, Toby still gained forty pounds during the pregnancy. She did not, fortunately, develop diabetes like her mother, perhaps because she was still so young.

Her son, Brett, was born vaginally. Toby's labor was prolonged, but Dr. Lightman stuck with her. Brett weight 8 pounds and 5 ounces, a normal healthy baby. Toby breast-fed Brett for ten months hoping that the nursing would help her lose weight. It may have helped some, but her inactivity and persistent hunger got the better of her.

CHAPTER SEVEN

# Answers to Common Questions

We've covered a lot of information in the last six chapters, and you may have some questions or need a review of certain points. Let's look at some typical questions and their answers.

**Dr. Anchors, are you saying that the main cause of obesity is a biochemical defect in the appestat in the brain? Does that mean that obesity is genetic?**

The tendency to obesity is certainly genetic. There is nothing more certain in the world. The weights of identical twins remain nearly identical throughout life, while the weights of non-identical twins are more often different. Overweight people tend to have overweight parents and overweight children. My favorite study of Nature vs. Nurture is the Danish study of adopted children. It turns out that the weights of the adopted children, after they grow up, correlate very well with the weights of their biological parents, and bear little relationship with the weights of their adoptive parents.

**But Dr. Anchors, my father is not overweight and my children aren't overweight!**

That doesn't disprove the thesis. If you mate a brown dog with a white dog, you get brown dogs, white dogs, and some dogs with spots. That doesn't mean that coat color in dogs is not genetic. It simply means that there is some variability in the expression of coat genes. There is variability in the expression of the "fat genes" too. By the way, some of your children may become overweight later.

**Does that mean that the defect in the appestat can be acquired?**

I don't know. I have stated that overweight people overeat because their appestat is insensitive to leptin. And I have stated that the defect in the appestat can be inherited. I have not said that the defect in the appestat can't also be acquired, later in life, because I don't know. Maybe it can. But whether the problem in the appestat is inherited or acquired, it's still true that the most certain way to fix the problem is to use appetite-suppressing drugs.

**Why are more and more Americans becoming obese each year? If the tendency to obesity is only genetic, how could the prevalence of obesity increase so fast?**

I didn't say that the tendency to obesity was *only* genetic. I said that the tendency is mainly a result of defective biochemistry in the brain, but that does not mean other factors don't play a role. Obviously, the number of people with a defective obesity gene can't be increasing as fast as the national average body weight. Other factors must be responsible. We know what some of them are:

- Increasing affluence of the population, which allows the following behavior . . .
  - Decreased exercise. People can afford more labor saving-devices. Fewer people are involved in manufacturing jobs that entail physical exercise, and more are involved in desk jobs. To afford better, more expensive labor-saving devices, people work longer hours than they used to. They have little time for scheduled aerobic exercise.
  - Restaurant owners and food producers package food in larger portions, so they can charge a higher price and collect a greater profit. Have you seen the size of a Snickers bar lately? People tend to eat the whole portion they purchased, hungry or not, rather than waste money. Not many dogs get anything in their doggy bags.

**Can the problem in the appestat resolve on its own, say if an obese patient continues on a voluntary, low-cal diet for a long time?**

Maybe so, but if you are depriving yourself month after month following the diet, I would suggest it's not worth the struggle. You are overlooking the chemical component (the appestat), which can be treated chemically (with appetite suppressants) and open the way for you to enjoy a less restricted life.

**I get hungry around the time of my menstrual period. Is it okay to take an appetite suppressant only during that time?**

If it works, do it. But let your doctor know what you are doing. I have some patients on maintenance therapy who take their medicines only before their menstrual period, but generally those trying to lose a lot of weight have to take the medicines all the time.

**I am not really hungry when I eat. Could it be that I eat out of nervousness?**

Some people do eat munchies as a nervous habit, but usually the true underlying drive is hunger. If munchers were really engaging in simple nervous eating, it wouldn't matter whether they ate high-fat or low-fat snacks. But the fact is they specifically buy high-cal snacks—they are both nervous *and* hungry.

An interesting experiment was described in *Scientific American* years ago, in which rats were subjected to electric shocks to make them nervous. The rats were then offered a choice of foods to eat. The scientists anticipated the rats would choose high-calorie foods over other types of food. What the scientists found, however, was that the rats preferred foods they had to chew for a long time, whether the foods were high-calorie or not.

For nervous patients on phen-Prozac, I recommend that they have bowls of chewable fruits and veggies available to satisfy their urge to munch. The patients on phen-Prozac will be satisfied with this, because their hunger has been controlled.

**My doctor will only give me phen-fen or Redux, saying there isn't enough published on phen-Prozac yet. Should I accept phen-fen?**

It depends on how ill you are. If obesity poses an immediate threat to your health, I think you should take phen-fen or Redux, if it is the only therapy available to you. The risk of PPH by my most pessimistic calculations is 1:10,000. If you are at mortal risk from obesity, and phen-fen or Redux is the only thing available, I say the benefits of these medications outweigh their risk of PPH. It won't be long before more physicians are prescribing phen-Prozac and you will have a safer option.

If your level of obesity is not an immediate health threat, you can afford to wait a year or two until you can find a doctor willing to prescribe phen-Prozac. In the meantime, try a voluntary diet and exercise program. I knew of one patient who went to one doctor and complained of depression, which she did not have, and another doctor to complain of overweight. She got Prozac from the first doctor and phentermine from the second, and took the two medicines together. Please, don't do this. It's not technically illegal, but it is much better to work with your doctor.

**If my doctor is unwilling to prescribe any form of medical appetite suppressant therapy, where can I find a doctor who will?**

If you live in a small town, it may be difficult in the next few years to find a physician who will prescribe medical appetite-suppressant therapy. People living in big cities can usually find a physician to prescribe appetite suppressants easily enough. This is because there are so many physicians in urban areas, there is a higher likelihood that a number of them will hold a favorable view of appetite suppressant therapy. This book and my article in *Archives of Internal Medicine* represent an effort to inform more doctors of the merits of phen-Prozac, but you must not be overly frustrated if your doctor doesn't jump right in. Doctors are naturally cautious people, and it is good that they are. Too often in the past, new medicines have appeared on the market, touted by their manufacturers, only to be withdrawn when a serious hazard was later discovered. Your physician is only thinking of your welfare in awaiting developments in the obesity field.

Work with your doctor to educate yourselves and share information so that you can undertake the appropriate obesity therapy for your condition, with mutual understanding and confidence.

You may contact Comprehensive Weight Loss Clinics at 310/444-6222, which can refer you to doctors in all fifty states who prescribe phen-fen (and, I hope, phen-Prozac soon), or call the Jenny Craig organization in your area.

You may also find a physician in your area willing to use drugs in the treatment of obesity by calling the American Society of Bariatric Physicians at 303/770-2526. Bariatric physicians are physicians who specialize in the treatment of obesity.

**My insurance plan won't pay for phentermine beyond thirty days, because it is "against FDA regulations." What can I do?**

Most insurance plans won't pay for phentermine at all. Most plans specifically do not cover medical treatment for obesity. You can hardly blame them; until now, there were no long-term effective medical therapies for obesity, but there were plenty of expensive, ineffective ones. Insurance companies define obesity as a "cosmetic problem" to escape the requirement to pay for treatment. Even if a morbidly obese patient can prove that the disease is not cosmetic, insurance companies can avoid payment by claiming that medical therapy is "experimental."

Prozac is the expensive component, not phentermine, and most insurance plans will pay for Prozac. Phentermine costs $17 for a six-week supply. That's 37 cents per day, about the cost of an aspirin, and most people can cover that expense.

FDA "regulations" on the use of phentermine past thirty days is ballyhoo. There are some voluntary FDA guidelines, but no mandatory regulations.

**Should I insist on brand-name forms of phentermine and Prozac, or will a generic form suffice?**

There are three brand-name forms of phentermine: Adipex, Fastin, and Ionamin. All three are significantly more expensive than the generic product and offer no real advantage for most people. Ionamin, a slow-release form, is popular with physicians because it avoids the nervousness and tremor that often attend phentermine prescribed initially in a full dose. Patients who start directly on 30 mg of phentermine often complain of nervousness in the middle of the day. This is especially true if they drink coffee with caffeine. The nervousness nearly always goes away after five days, even when the drug is continued, but many patients stop the drug before the side effect has time to subside. Some physicians prescribe Ionamin to get around this problem, but there is a more economical way: start phentermine in a dose of 15 mg for a week before progressing to 30 mg, and drink decaffeinated coffee while using phentermine.

Prozac will not be available as a generic drug until the year 2002. Of all the SSRI drugs that work combined with phentermine, only trazodone is available as a generic.

This issue is really too complex to work out by yourself. Make your doctor aware of your concerns about cost when she is writing your prescriptions. She will find the least expensive way, based on current medical therapeutics and economics.

**Are there any good substitutes for phentermine in combination with an SSRI?**

Tenuate can be used in place of phentermine. It is not quite as strong, but that might be an advantage for patients who are especially sensitive to the stimulant side effects of phentermine.

**Are there any substitutes for Prozac in combination with phentermine?**

Yes, many. I mentioned that Zoloft, trazodone, and Luvox seem to work as well as Prozac.

- Luvox is a good choice for patients whose sex drive is reduced by Prozac.
- Zoloft is a good choice for patients on medications for other conditions, because it interferes least with the metabolism of other drugs. Zoloft is good, too, if the phentermine causes too much constipation; Zoloft loosens stools.
- Trazodone is available as a cheap generic drug, and it helps patients sleep.

Nevertheless, patients and physicians should be aware that I have much more experience with phen-Prozac than with any other combination.

**Are there medicines other than appetite suppressants available to deal with obesity?**

Xenical, a product of Hoffman-LaRoche, will be released in late 1997. It interferes with the absorption of dietary fat in the intestines. Significant weight loss has been achieved in studies with Xenical, but the medicine tends to produce greasy stools and diarrhea. Dietary fat not absorbed in the gut naturally finds its way to the stool. I have no experience with Xenical and don't want to judge it until I have had a chance to try it on some patients. But I have a moral objection to it. It upsets me to think of giving overweight Americans a medicine to block the absorption of food, when so many children are starving in the world.

Some years ago trials were done with medicines that blocked the absorption of starch. These were quickly withdrawn because they caused excessive bloating and diarrhea. They were ineffective as well, because the major portion of calories in the food overweight people eat is in fat, not starch.

Olestra is not a medicine, but is a new kind of cooking oil that is not absorbed by the body and contains no calories. Many diet foods, chips, and pretzels, are cooked in Olestra; the bags are marked with the word. Rarely, people have complained of gastrointestinal distress from these products, but more often than not they are well tolerated.

Combination appetite suppressant therapy addresses the problem at its source. Reducing the calorie content of food, or reducing the absorption of food, only means that the obese person will need to eat more food to get rid of hunger. Remember the appestat!

**Should I take vitamins while I am following your weight-loss program?**

No special vitamin supplements need to be taken. The reason this question is sometimes asked is because, in the past, patients following extremely low-calorie diets or taking liquid protein supplements were advised to take vitamin supplements to supply vitamins missing in the food. Because patients on phen-Prozac eat balanced diets of regular food, vitamins aren't missing.

Everyone, thin or fat, dieting or not, should take the antioxidant vitamins C and E, because these particular vitamins have proven helpful in preventing heart disease and cancer. Strict vegetarians should take vitamin B-12 supplements, or supplement their diet with yeast, because vitamin B-12 is low in vegetables.

**If I get to a plateau on phen-Prozac and cannot lose any more weight, can Redux be added to the medical program? Vice versa, if I am taking phen-fen, can Prozac be added to fenfluramine, rather than substituted?**

There are no easy answers to these questions at this time. The *PDR* contains strong warnings regarding simultaneous use of two serotonin-active medicines, such as Prozac and fenfluramine. There have been reports of a moderately rare "serotonin syndrome" resulting from this practice, involving agitation, sleeplessness, fast heartbeat, and tremor.

Dr. Richard Rothman has prescribed fenfluramine and Prozac together for some patients with no apparent negative consequences.[1] Some patients were able to lose weight, who failed on ordinary doses of phen-fen or phen-Prozac.

Until the combined use of fenfluramine and Prozac has been extensively investigated, fenfluramine should not be used together with an SSRI. Two SSRIs may be used together, as long as the doses are kept low. I sometimes combine low-dose Prozac with low-dose trazodone in depressed patients, if needed, because trazodone helps people sleep.

**Do you always start obese patients on phentermine and Prozac, or do you sometimes start with another combination?**

I only start patients on appetite suppressant therapy if: 1) they have failed on previous voluntary diets, 2) their body mass index (BMI) is over 30, or they have adverse consequences of obesity and their BMI is over 27, and 3) they have no contraindications to the therapy. And, yes, I do start most patients on phen-Prozac, because I have the most confidence and experience with that combination.

In certain situations, I use other SSRI medications. For example, if the patient had preexisting depression and was in good balance on an antidepressant known to be one that works for weight loss, I would stick with the patient's current antidepressant.

If the patient already has a problem with insomnia, I recommend phentermine in the morning and 50 to 100 mg of trazodone at night, instead of Prozac. Phen-trazodone works, and trazodone allows people to sleep in a pattern of natural deep sleep.

If the patient complains of a low sex drive, Luvox at 25 to 50 mg is a better choice than Prozac, which can suppress the sex drive in some individuals. More often it causes a delay in orgasm, which can actually be an advantage in some men.

If the patient complains of chronic constipation, I would use Zoloft because it has a tendency to cause diarrhea, which offsets the tendency of phentermine to induce constipation.

**I started taking phentermine once before, several years ago, and became very agitated. I couldn't keep taking it. Am I going to be even more nervous if I take phentermine and Prozac together?**

You could be, but I haven't seen much of this. At the beginning of therapy, I start patients on a low dose of phentermine to give the brain time to adapt. Sometimes I write a prescription for 15-mg generic phentermine capsules, but more often I show patients how to open the 30-mg capsule and discard half the contents. Or I have patients take one-fourth of the 30-mg dose the first day, one-third the next, one-half the next, and so on, up to the full dose after a week. Nearly everyone can tolerate this gradual approach.

The fact that the brain adapts to the phentermine does not mean that the patient has become addicted to the medicine; generally the same dose will keep working, and there are no significant withdrawal effects upon stopping the medicine.

The side effects of phentermine are not enhanced by combination with Prozac. The dose of Prozac used for weight loss—10 mg or so—is so much lower than the dose normally used for depression, it is unlikely that severe anxiety reactions will occur in a weight-loss patient.

**I was taking phen-fen from another doctor and did not have much success. Should I try phen-Prozac?**

If you did not lose weight with phen-fen, you may lose weight slowly or not at all on phen-Prozac, but it is still worth a try. Seven of my patients did not lose weight on phen-Prozac even when they did everything I asked. But that was seven out of nearly six hundred! A few dozen patients did not lose weight or lost slowly, because they did not take the medicines as I prescribed them or they ate when they weren't hungry or failed to exercise. They cannot be counted as treatment failures, because they did not follow the treatment program. Some patients who were not successful with phen-fen were successful with phen-Prozac.

The success rate of phen-Prozac for my patients has been higher than the reported success rate claimed for any other appetite suppressant program, but it is not 100 percent. I believe that phen-Prozac works more consistently than phen-fen, but I'll be the first to mention that I have not had much experience with phen-fen. I don't prescribe fenfluramine because it entails an unnecessary risk of PPH.

I believe that both phen-fen and phen-Prozac work better than Redux. It stands to reason—Redux, a form of fenfluramine, is only one component of the phen-fen combination. One would not expect it to work better than the full combination. I have seen a large number of patients who failed on Redux but have lost weight successfully and continuously on phen-Prozac.

Dr. George Bray and Dr. John Foreyt have delivered a series of lectures around the country at the behest of the Wyeth-Ayerst company, makers of Redux, in which the doctors seem to be lowering expectations for appetite suppressant therapy.[2] They insist that many obese patients will not respond to appetite suppressant therapy. Those who do not get a good response in the first few weeks of therapy, they claim, are doomed to failure. I have great respect for these two doctors, but I think their opinion has been colored by their experience with Redux. I have had good results with phen-Prozac.

**Can I stop taking phen-Prozac at any time? Will it hurt me to stop? How should I stop taking it?**

You can stop taking the medicine at any time. I normally have patients stop as they approach ideal body weight. This allows us to see if the appestat has reset so that they can stay off the medication permanently. But patients can stop therapy whenever they want. In particular, there is no need to take the medication during religious fasts or when you are sick, because you are not going to eat much on those days anyway. There are no withdrawal symptoms. Once the patient is off the medicine too long, the patient may gain back weight.

**What happens when I reach my ideal body weight?**

Your doctor will stop the medicines to see if your body will maintain its new weight. About 25 percent of patients stay more or less at the same weight and won't need to take the medication any longer. A few, after a year or so, drift upward and need a refresher course, but generally they have been "cured" of obesity.

The other 75 percent regain weight after they stop taking the medicine. Such patients need maintenance therapy, which I describe as the lowest dose in the least frequency that keeps their weight constant. Usually, this means about 15 mg of phentermine and 10 mg of Prozac every other day for some weeks of the month. Patients learn to be savvy about when they need their medications. They call in for refills as needed and keep me advised of their weight. I see them for regular but not frequent follow-ups.

**What is the best way to introduce my doctor to the subject of weight-loss therapy with phen-Prozac?**

Show your doctor Chapter 12 of this book, which I've written directly to doctors, and introduce the topic by writing or saying something like the following:

Dear Doctor,

I respect you for your medical knowledge and your honest concern for my health and safety. Please accord me the same respect by believing me when I tell you that I have followed your diet and exercise advice in the past, yet in spite of it I have not been able to lose weight. Recent research has demonstrated that obesity is largely determined by biochemical factors in the brain, rather than by bad habits or character flaws. Therefore, diet and exercise alone are unlikely to succeed on a long-term basis. There are medicines available now that reduce weight by reducing appetite, and these medicines have been shown to be both safe and effective in long-term trials. My body mass index is over 30; I am at increased risk for a number of serious obesity-related diseases. My obesity is at least as dangerous to me as high blood pressure would be, and should be treated equally as seriously.

I would like to take combination appetite suppressant therapy to supplement my continued efforts at diet and exercise. You can read about combination appetite suppressant therapy in the article by Dr. Michael Weintraub in *Clinical Pharmacological Therapeutics* 51(5): 581–646 (1992), and in the book *Safer Than Phen-Fen!* by Dr. Anchors. Doctor Anchors has also written an article in *Archives of Internal Medicine,* 157:1270 (1997) titled "Fluoxetine Is a Safer Alternative to Fenfluramine in the Medical Treatment of Obesity." The best-tolerated initial approach to therapy is a combination of phentermine and either Prozac or Zoloft. Both Pondimin and Redux can cause primary pulmonary hypertension and heart valve disease, and I don't want to take that risk.

Thank you for listening.

Sincerely yours,

____________

# Toby's Story

**PART 7**

I MET TOBY when her son, Brett, was three years old. Toby's weight was up to 280 pounds. She was an officer at her bank, but she had to take frequent time off for illness. She was a valued asset to her employers, but they were seriously worried about her health. She had trouble moving around in the bank, often scraping herself against the desks, and once she got stuck in the door of the vault. She always seemed to be out of breath.

Frank's weight was 264 at the time, and he had developed sleep apnea. Many of the nights he stayed late at the office were because he could not finish his work during the day. But when he stayed late, he often fell asleep at his desk. He hid the traffic tickets he had received for driving erratically. He had cracked up their car several times after falling asleep at the wheel.

Toby wanted to have another baby, but knew she dared not try to get pregnant at her weight. The couple was having sex rarely, although they loved each other very much. They were both exhausted much of the time, and the effort was almost too great.

Toby's mother, Christina, had died of ovarian cancer and complications of diabetes at age fifty. Toby worried that she was a prime candidate for diabetes and couldn't imagine living on such a restricted diet.

I explained to Toby in very clinical terms that obesity has a biochemical basis in the brain—that obese people are persistently hungry because their appetite thermostat in their brain does not respond to the hormone leptin properly. Somehow, the combination of phentermine and Prozac makes that better, and the patients on phen-Prozac continue to lose weight. They feel satisfied with less food and their hunger drive returns to that of a person with a normal appetite thermostat. I would still expect her to make a good faith effort to choose low-calorie foods, and she needed to get daily exercise, but with the medicines she would have success.

As I explained to Toby the actual cause for her obesity—that it was a disease—I saw her shoulders lift and her eyes brighten. She was filled with hope because I was telling her something different from the routine, something more closely related to her actual experience of life. She wasn't stupid; she had figured out for herself that obesity had more to do with hunger than with bad habits, but so many of her friends and doctors had told her otherwise that she was afraid to profess her belief. She listened to me with great relief.

Toby told me about her previous negative experience with the side effects of Ionamin, a brand of phentermine. I assured her that she would have a better experience with phentermine, because we would start it up slowly. I also explained that the reason she had stopped losing weight on Ionamin was because it was only half the formula. Her prescription card would pay for the Prozac. She had to pay $17 for a six-week supply of generic phentermine.

When Toby returned after six weeks, she had already lost 20 pounds. She had no side effects other than dry mouth. It was summer and she complained of some increased sweating, but none of the side effects bothered her. Mostly, she wanted to tell me how good she felt.

Frank came with her on the next visit. He wanted to try the medicine, too. He had a referral from his primary care doctor, who had been grappling with Frank's sleep apnea. Frank wore a mask on his face at night, through which a thin stream of air was blown into his nostrils. The apparatus, called CPAP, had reduced his symptoms of sleep apnea, but his physician wanted him to lose weight to eliminate the source of the sleep apnea. Frank worked out at the gym every morning before work, but the extra activity only increased his hunger. He had not lost a pound.

Six weeks later on the third visit for Toby and the second for Frank, both spouses had lost more weight: thirteen pounds for Toby and seventeen pounds for Frank. Toby was feeling sexier, chomping at the bit to start the next baby. Frank had found that the Prozac reduced his sex drive somewhat, so I switched his Prozac to Luvox.

After a year of treatment, at the writing of this book, Toby has lost ninety-six pounds, and she is pregnant with her second baby. Frank has lost fifty pounds. His sleep apnea has resolved. He no longer wears the mask at night.

Both people lost weight faster at first. The rate of weight loss slowed down after a few months, but they have continued to shed pounds. Toby has to be off the medicines while she is pregnant; she will resume them after the baby is born. She recently told me she was getting some good exercise from the dance class she and Frank were taking together. She also told me she had been accepted to a great business school and would be starting after the baby was born.

Both Frank and Toby are likely to continue to lose weight on the medicines. If they were in the group that goes into a plateau, they would have done so already. Because neither has,

I don't think either will. Phen-Prozac and phen-Luvox are ideal for them. They will reach their ideal body weight or near enough to it for them to have normal, healthy lives. Just as I continue to give medicine year after year to my patients with high blood pressure, I will continue to give Frank and Toby the medicines to keep their weight low, if necessary, for the rest of their lives. This is, after all, what medicine is for.

Chronic diseases like obesity increase the chances of other serious health problems and ultimately shorten lives. But the insidious part of the disease is that it steals bits and pieces of lives in the process. As a doctor, when I find a treatment that not only stops the ravages of the disease, but gives back to my patients the quality of their lives—well, it doesn't get any better than that.

CHAPTER EIGHT

# Don't Be Afraid of Food

I used to tell my patients to eat like the people in Sri Lanka or India. I urged them to eat fruits and vegetables, like people in China and Vietnam. I thought they would lose weight this way. All foods, I declared, were composed of only three ingredients that matter in terms of calories: fats, carbohydrates, and proteins.

**Calorie Content of Dietary Components[1]**

| | |
|---|---|
| carbohydrate | 4 calories per gram |
| protein | 4 calories per gram |
| fat | 9 calories per gram |

It can be seen from the table on page 125 that if people concentrate on high-carbohydrate foods and cut back on fat intake, they will automatically reduce their calorie intake.[2,3] I told my patients that people in Third World countries eat mainly high-carbohydrate foods, such as rice and beans. Consequently, I said, one rarely sees overweight people in those countries.

I thought I was clever until some of my patients, who came from Sri Lanka and Vietnam, challenged me. "Hold on!" they said. "We have overweight people in our country. They're not as overweight as overweight Americans, to be sure, but there are almost as many."

I was shocked. I didn't believe it until I confirmed their stories by referring to World Health Organization statistics in the 1995 *World Almanac.*

I should not have been so surprised. There are just as many people in Asian countries whose appestat is resistant to leptin as there are in the United States. These folks become overweight, relative to their population, eating large amounts of rice and pickles. If the appestat-leptin system is working properly, people can stay lean eating at McDonald's (this is not to say that they will be healthy; read on). But if their appestats are out of whack, even Optifast and Lean Cuisine won't keep them thin. People always, eventually, eat until they are no longer hungry; at that point, those with a defective appestat have eaten too much.

The only way to control weight is to control hunger. Diet advocates from Oprah Winfrey to Nathan Pritikin have focused on the fact that obese people snack on high-fat foods, but that observation is useless in defining a successful long-term weight-control strategy because the fundamental problem faced by overweight people is excessive hunger, not ignorance. To persist in telling people that if they would only give up ice cream and chips their weight problem would be solved merely exposes the ignorance of the nutritionist. Overweight people don't eat high-fat foods because they are stupid or lazy, but because they are hungry. They know that high-fat foods satisfy their hunger best. They know that carrot sticks won't do the job. I see tears in their eyes when I voice this opinion; a doctor finally understands them.

---

*The only way to control weight is to control hunger.*

---

When this awareness that weight loss is not dependent on what type of food one eats began to dawn on me, it seemed so revolutionary that I had to try it out on myself. For one year, from April 1996 to April 1997, I ate every breakfast at McDonald's and every lunch at Burger King, being careful to eat only when I was hungry and to stop when I was full. I did not gain weight! I weighed 176 pounds when I started, and 176 pounds when I finished. I am 5'10" tall and no one in my family has ever been obese. We just don't have the gene(s) for obesity; our appestats function normally.

That is not to say that eating more fruit and vegetables is not a good thing to do for a number of other health-related reasons! During my year of eating burgers and biscuits, my cholesterol level climbed, my blood pressure went up, and I developed a kidney stone. There is direct evidence that vegetarians live longer, thin or fat.[4] There is an enormous amount of literature on the need for fiber in the diet, and there are a zillion nutrients in plants that promote good health.

## Dietary Guidelines for Health and Weight Loss

When I prescribe phen-Prozac to patients, my basic advice regarding food is simple: don't eat when you are not hungry and stop eating when you are full. Usually that is all I have to say.

If the subsequent weight loss is slow or they hit a plateau, I go a few steps further. I advise them to cease eating desserts, and I inquire into their alcohol consumption. I often strike gold with the women in the former respect, and the men in the latter.

### Obey the Eight Commandments

If pressed further, I will provide a few more pieces of advice on the subject of diet. Here are what I call the Eight Commandments.

1. Don't eat when you are not hungry. Eat slowly, and stop eating when you are full.
2. Don't buy what you shouldn't eat.
3. Eat your largest meal in the middle of the day.
4. Fill your plate with low-calorie side dishes first. Only when you have eaten a full plate of these items should you venture to fill your plate with the main course.
5. Cut back on foods that come from land animals.

6. Eat foods that are spicier and more aromatic.
7. Don't eat in restaurants so often. When you do eat out, choose restaurants that serve smaller portions or share dishes.
8. If you are drinking too much alcohol, cut back or get help.

Let's consider the commandments one at a time.

1. *Don't eat when you are not hungry. Eat slowly, and stop eating when you are full.*

An ancient Zen proverb says that the true path to happiness is "to eat when hungry and sleep when sleepy." Sounds too simple to be true, but think how miserable you have been when you did not obey this advice. The appestat tells you only when you need to eat, and phen-Prozac suppresses only the appestat. If you eat even when you are not hungry, you are bypassing the signals of your appestat and even phen-Prozac won't salvage the situation.

Previously I said that I ate every meal at a McDonald's or a Burger King for a year and did not gain weight. That was not entirely true. For a few months in the middle of that period, I got into the habit of eating bags of Hershey's Kisses. During that time, I did gain a little weight. It was a stupid habit—I was not eating the Kisses out of hunger—and when I realized that I was gaining weight, I cut out the Kisses. Without making any other changes in my diet and exercise pattern, my weight declined to its previous level.

I used to think that most of the eating by obese people was of the Hershey's Kiss type. I changed my mind when I saw how many people lost weight with phen-Prozac, without being specifically counseled on diet. It must be that the main factor in obesity is hunger-driven eating, not boredom- or stress-driven snacking. It's the only way to explain why phen-Prozac works so well.

Dr. Mark Eig suggested to me that Kiss-eating is a form of obsessive-compulsive behavior, suppressed by the Prozac in the phen-Prozac combination, but I don't think that is correct: the dose of Prozac in phen-Prozac is too low to have that effect. The doses of Prozac used for clinical OCD are much higher. I think the Prozac in the phen-Prozac combination has a direct effect in enhancing the effect of phentermine on the appestat.

I am not saying that obese people never engage in stress-eating or eating out of boredom. I am not saying that the recreational eating they do is not a problem. I am only saying that recreational eating it is not the most important element in obesity. Anyone who claims that Dr. Anchors says "It doesn't matter what you eat" is distorting the truth.

Another reason why people eat when they are not hungry is the compulsion to "clean the plate." Men might feel that they have wasted money if food is left on the table. Women may worry that they have deprived starving children in Biafra if they don't eat every last bit. But look at the situation logically. The money is already spent; Dick won't be a dollar richer if he eats the rest of the pot roast, and Jane won't help Biafran children by eating the dessert she didn't really want. The trick is, buy less, cook less, use more Tupperware. That will save money and indirectly help the children in Biafra.

It is very important, when you are eating, to eat slowly, so that you can tell when you are full. This will spare you from going beyond "full" and arriving at "stuffed." I remember sleeping over at my friend Bobby's house when I was a boy. Bobby and his family were obese; I recognize that fact in retrospect. My family and I were thin, and we were used to talking at the dinner table. Dinner was the social hour at my house—the only time when the whole family was together.

Bobby's family, on the other hand, didn't talk at the table. Instead, for ten minutes after the food hit the table, there was nothing said but "pass this" and "pass that," and the only sounds were those of scooping, scraping, gulping, and chewing. I suffered culture shock the night I ate at Bobby's house. Only after everything had been eaten did anyone venture to talk.

People who eat rapidly cannot possibly know when they have reached the point of being full. Phen-Prozac won't correct this dysfunctional habit. Obese patients have to take charge of their manner of eating. They must learn to eat slowly, to savor, to chew, and to converse. Medicines can only do so much; some aspects of obesity are under voluntary control.

2. *Don't buy what you shouldn't eat.*

It seems blindingly obvious, but it is worth saying, that you can't eat what you don't buy. It is also true that if you buy something, you will probably eat it. Generally it is easier to restrain the urge to buy high-calorie foods in the store than it is to resist the urge to eat the stuff once it is in your home. You are in the grocery store for only thirty minutes. A bag of Hershey's Kisses in your pantry will tempt you day after day: I have learned from experience.

Most people eat almost all their meals from the same list of ten or twelve dishes that they have learned to prepare. People seldom consult cookbooks to plan family meals. How many of your cookbooks have even been opened since you bought them? How many have even one tomato stain on them?

The usual reason cited for such culinary conservatism is that there isn't time, or there isn't money, or the kids won't eat anything new. These are facts of life.

But when you are trying to lose weight it is important to look over your standard repertory of dishes to see if there are any dishes that are especially high in fat and calories. Find a different way to prepare the dish, or find a different dish altogether that is more healthful.

3. *Eat your largest meal in the middle of the day.*

This one is not so obvious, and it is not convenient. The average, busy American skips breakfast and eats a hurried lunch. When the American finally gets home, he or she wants to relax and eat. When I used to collect diet records from patients, it was not unusual to find that they consumed 90 percent of their daily calories at supper.

Eating at night is absolutely the worst time to eat if you are trying to lose weight. There is a biological clock in your pancreas that determines that your pancreas puts out the most insulin of the day around 7 o'clock in the evening. One of the major effects of insulin is that it encourages the tissues to store food as fat.

*Eating at night is absolutely the worst time to eat if you are trying to lose weight.*

It is far better to consume the main meal of the day at lunch, or to divide the calories between breakfast and lunch. Elsewhere in the world people eat like this. In many European and Latin countries, shopkeepers close their shops at midday and go home for lunch. After lunch, they take a siesta.

In addition to avoiding the peak of insulin output, moving the main meal to midday allows phen-Prozac to work better. Patients who take phentermine at sun up, but eat a big meal at 7 o'clock at night are expecting the appetite-suppressing power of phentermine to last all day until supper, and then wear off by bedtime, so they can sleep—it is too much to ask. If they eat their largest meal at lunch instead, the phentermine can do a better job of reducing excess hunger.

4. *Fill your plate with low-calorie side dishes first. Only when you have eaten a full plate of these should you venture to fill your plate with the main course.*

As I have watched American families eat, I have noticed that women tend to eat salad first, then soup, when it's available, then vegetables, then the main course. Come to think of it, that's the way my mother taught me to eat!

During all this, they are having a conversation. Following the order of the meal and talking slows the eating down and permits them to tell when they are full.

Most men I have observed go straight for the main dish, usually the highest-calorie, most hunger-quenching item on the table. Attacking the beef when they are at the peak of their hunger results in eating too much beef before the brain realizes what has happened. Moreover, filling up on beef and cheese, they eat less grains, veggies, and beans, and miss important nutrients. It's a fact that most peas and carrots served to men end up in the garbage disposal.

Eating side dishes first, before the main course, reduces overall calorie consumption. The meal is just as satisfying, and more healthful. I knew there was a reason to listen to my mother!

5. *Cut back on foods that come from land animals.*

My patients with obesity, diabetes, gout, high cholesterol, and high blood pressure, in other words nearly all of them, love to ask me what they should eat. There is a strong tendency in most societies to believe that most of our ills are a result of what we eat. I believe that most of what happens to us is a result of our genes, but the "what-we-eat" theory is more comforting to people, because it gives them something they can do to help themselves.

I don't want to spend a lot of time during office visits going into the details of calorie counts and food exchanges, so I have come up with simple rules patients could follow. Reminding myself that fat has 9 calories per gram and carbohydrate and protein have only 4 calories per gram, the simplest rule I can come up with is to tell people to eat less food from land animals. This tactic cuts down on the intake of saturated fat, lowers blood cholesterol a little, and reduces the intake of dietary DNA so there is less tendency to gout. There is less fat—that helps diabetics. Since high-fat foods tend to be high-salt foods, eating less food from land animals reduces salt intake, reducing high blood pressure. No other rule so succinctly describes a healthful diet.

6. *Eat foods that are spicier and more aromatic.*

You will eat less, and be more satisfied, if the food you eat is more heavily spiced and aromatic. I have no documentation for this, but I know it to be true, from observation of people and from comparing cuisines of different cultures.

7. *Don't eat in restaurants so often. When you do eat out, choose restaurants that serve smaller portions or share dishes.*

Americans spend 44 percent of their food budget in restaurants. We are busy, on the go. We have little time to shop and cook. We want to enjoy the "good life." The good life, for most people, means eating in restaurants. How can we do it without busting our calorie budget?

If you have a choice, French restaurants are a good deal. They serve small servings of delicious food on large pretty plates and charge a pretty price. Just don't stick around for dessert! Japanese restaurants are ideal for dieting gourmets; they serve a pea pod at the bottom of a bowl of hot water, call it soup, and charge $50; you're not likely to overeat. Do as the Romans do in Italian restaurants: eat noodles with tomato or pesto sauce; stay away from Alfredo sauce. Seafood restaurants are good, as long as you avoid butter and tartar sauce. Chinese, Vietnamese, and Thai restaurants are nice. Mexican restaurants are a caloric wipe-out; save them for a birthday or Cinco de Mayo.

It's hard to know what to say about fast-food restaurants. Few people over the age of ten enjoy fast-food restaurants for their own sake, but where else can you eat so quickly and cheaply? With a little foresight, people could bring a lunch box to work, but the foods most people put in lunch boxes are not much better than fast food. How many types of low-fat sandwich can you name? And the stuff in lunch boxes is so cold.

I have often said that if the U.S. Department of Health wanted to do something to improve the health of Americans, the most cost-effective thing they could do would be to subsidize a chain of good, low-fat restaurants in convenient places! It's not such a crazy idea. Wouldn't you like to be able to eat a healthful lunch while running errands at the post office?

8. *If you are drinking too much alcohol, cut back or get help.*

It's an ugly secret that every family physician knows: alcohol is a major cause of obesity in America. Alcohol counts for 7 calories per milliliter, or about 200 calories per ounce. A 12-ounce beer has 150 calories—about the same as a glass of wine or a shot of liquor.

---

*It's an ugly secret that every family physician knows: alcohol is a major cause of obesity in America.*

---

Beer calories are especially likely to cause obesity because beer itself does nothing to satisfy hunger. The obese beer drinker still overeats, on top of all the calories from beer. I have heard people speculate that the obesity observed in beer drinkers—the "beer belly"—is a consequence of biochemical effects on the liver. Baloney! It's a direct consequence of too many calories going in.

The U.S. population drinks an average of 32 gallons of beer per adult per year,[5] which, as horrible as it sounds, is only the tenth highest consumption in the world. The people in the nine countries that consume more beer than we do get more exercise than we do; they are not as fat as you might expect, but they still have a problem with obesity.

Thirty-two gallons of beer per adult works out to 280 calories a day! It's hard to see how we would ever trim the national waistline without cutting back on beer. And I haven't even mentioned wine and hard liquor!

## A Smorgasbord of Thoughts About Meals

Though your choices of food may not make all the difference in losing weight, given that you eat only to the point of feeling full, food does make a difference in treating other medical conditions and decreases your chance of becoming sick. All people should eat in a healthful manner.

On the next few pages are some pointers about preparing and eating food. It is true that most of the excess calories obese people consume are a consequence of excess hunger, but some of the calories they ingest are a consequence of simple errors in thinking that have nothing to do with hunger or enjoyable eating.

### Salad

If your doctor has put you on an appetite suppressant, you are no longer under the thumb of hunger. You have the leisure to enjoy salad. But it is important to know how to eat salad.

#### THE TYPICAL AMERICAN WRONG WAY

a bowl of iceberg lettuce evenly cut up = zero calories,
zero flavor
6 ounces dressing from a bottle, for flavor = 900 calories

#### THE HEALTHFUL, RIGHT WAY

Buy a number of different kinds of lettuce. America's grocers are putting many different types of lettuce out on their shelves these days. More Americans ought to be buying them. At one ordinary grocery store I was able to find: iceberg, romaine, endive, escarole, Boston, and red leaf lettuce. Lettuce is a great source of fiber and vitamin C.

Lettuce isn't the only leafy thing you can put in a salad. Add fresh spinach, cabbage, bok choy, parsley, leeks, watercress, and cilantro. The leaves of all these greens should be washed in water and pulled apart or cut in different sizes for variety and visual interest. Other items such as mushrooms, olives, beans, chickpeas, broccoli, cauliflower, and carrots can be added, too.

Salad should be assembled fresh in large batches or made ahead of time and stored in tight zipper-lock plastic bags. Do not add dressing before storing the salad, and don't add croutons in the bag; they'll get soggy. Don't add cheese either. It makes the salad in the bag sticky. As a matter of fact, don't add cheese to salad at all. Cheese adds calories and covers up the flavor of the greens.

For dinner, a portion of salad should be placed in a mixing bowl and tossed with a light coating of oil and vinegar. Pepper should be added at the table from a pepper mill, a little gadget that's worth the investment. Freshly ground pepper is so much more aromatic than preground pepper.

Don't use bottled dressings unless they are marked "nonfat." The ordinary commercial dressings on the shelf all have 110 (Italian) to 160 (Ranch) calories per 2-ounce serving, and I know perfectly well that the average American man, if he is going to eat salad at all, puts a lot more than 2 ounces of dressing on his salad!

### Bread

Some kind of bread should be eaten with every meal. Bread is the staff of life everywhere—except in America, where we use bread only as a convenient holder for sandwich meat.[6] A Frenchman's lunch is a loaf of bread and a glass of wine.

Many Americans think that bread is fattening. They are confused. A slice of Roman Meal bread—my favorite—contains only 60 calories and less than a gram of fat—and Roman Meal is not a low-calorie bread! White bread has no more calories than a piece of styrofoam.

I live in the Washington, D.C., area—a crossroad of cultures and a crossroad of bread. There is wonderful, dense German bread, bubbly French bread, dark Russian pumpernickel, tangy Jewish rye bread and challah, Syrian pita, and Afghan flat breads. The Indians make a hundred different kinds of pan bread. The Ethiopians don't use plates or silverware; they plop their food down on a large, round flat bread called *injera.* Diners tear off bits of injera and use it to snap up clumps of food: something red, something yellow—I never have any idea what I am eating in an Ethiopian restaurant. It's fun, and that is what mealtimes should be.

The key thing with bread is to eat the bread *al puro*—in its pure form. Don't cover it up with butter. Both butter and margarine are pure fat—9 calories per gram—and they disguise the subtle flavors of the bread.

### Cheese

Some of my obese patients, in the years before I discovered phen-Prozac, became vegetarians in an effort to lose weight. A few succeeded, a little, for a while. I questioned the ones who did not lose weight, because I wondered why the strategy had not worked for them. Some of them succumbed to the Hershey's Kiss syndrome (seen earlier); they were satisfying their hunger with chocolate. The other large group was abusing cheese. Many people think of cheese as low-fat. Cheese gets good PR in our society, and meat gets bad. But if you read the labels on cheese, you'll see it is very high in fat and calories. Generally the hard cheeses, such as Parmesan and Cheddar, are the worst, and the soft cheeses, such as cottage and ricotta, are better. Swiss cheese and mozzarella are intermediate. Cheese is never a diet bargain, but it is a good source of calcium and protein. The best way to use cheese is as a condiment, as a sprinkle or light dip. Dieters addicted to Roquefort or bleu cheese dressing would do better to add a little oil and vinegar to salad, and crumple a small block of bleu cheese on top. Bottled Roquefort dressing is 50 percent sour cream.

## Meat

I do not get into the red meat versus white meat issue with my patients because it doesn't matter. That's the truth! The fat content of red meat has come down so far in the last fifteen years, while the fat content of chicken and turkey has gone up, that it doesn't make any difference anymore. The Texas longhorn was almost extinct; the species was reduced to two herds in Texas kept for making Western movies. But look again! Over recent years, the longhorns have been vigorously bred because they furnish especially low-fat beef. Steers are being fed on the prairie again, instead of on corn. It would bring a sentimental tear to a cowboy's eye.

Patients who think they are losing weight or lowering their cholesterol level by eating white meat are fooling themselves. You can look at a piece of meat and tell whether it is fatty. So look! Don't be complacent just because the meat is white.

These days you can buy ground beef at the grocery store that has only 7 percent fat. If you want to make hamburgers, get the lowest-fat hamburger meat that you can find, and grill it so that the extra fat drips out. Cook the meat through, and never put the meat back on the same plate the meat occupied before being cooked; put cooked burgers on a fresh plate. This is to avoid contaminating cooked meat with bacteria present on the meat before it was cooked.

### French Fries

Yes, you can still eat french fries! The thing is to make your own and not cook them in oil; there is no need for that. Spread fries on a baking dish and bake them in the oven at 400°F until brown and crispy. French fries are not fattening when cooked in this way, and they taste fine. They taste even better if you season them with a mixture of celery salt, paprika, mustard, black pepper, laurel leaves, cloves, ginger, mace, and cardamom.

### Dessert

Don't eat dessert. You don't need it. Desserts are the most unnecessary, senseless, fattening things people eat. If you have followed my advice up to now and eaten the meal slowly in stages, you should feel pleasantly full. The phen-Prozac, if you're taking it, is suppressing your excess hunger; so why do you need dessert?

---

*The Western yen for dessert is a habit, pure and simple—a habit that must be broken!*

---

Dessert is a conceit of Western culture. The Chinese don't eat dessert at all. If you ask for the dessert menu in a Chinese restaurant, you are handed a little plastic tray with a fortune cookie and a check. The Western yen for dessert is a habit, pure and simple—a habit that must be broken!

If you are genuinely still hungry after supper, eat some more of the main course, have an espresso, or eat fruit.

If you find you are persistently hungry after supper, ask the doctor to raise your dose of appetite suppressant or consider taking the appetite suppressant later in the day. This will seldom be necessary. Most people are full by the time dessert is offered. It only takes a little self-restraint.

## Seasonings and Extras

### SALT

Many dieters seem concerned and confused about salt. Physicians often advise patients with high blood pressure to consume less salt, because blood pressure can be reduced in some patients by a low-salt diet, but this advice has nothing specifically to do with obesity.

When physicians say "salt," what they mean is "sodium chloride," a particular kind of salt that we know as "table salt." You can eat all the potassium chloride ("lite salt") you want and it will not raise your blood pressure, but potassium chloride doesn't taste very good. "Salt substitute" does not contain sodium or potassium; it's a spice.

Not all patients with high blood pressure respond to lowering the level of sodium in the diet. In such cases, the patient should move on to antihypertensive medicines.

Even though sodium itself has nothing to do with causing obesity, it is related to obesity in a couple of ways.

First, nearly all high-sodium foods are high-fat foods. Hence, any patient eating a high-sodium diet is assuredly eating a high-fat diet. Not a good move, if you are obese.

Second, if you are obese, overconsumption of sodium can lead to swollen ankles. The body content of sodium determines the total body content of fluid. If the body's sodium content is high, fluid tends to pool in the lowest area of the body—the legs—and the circulatory system has trouble getting the fluid back into circulation. The kidneys are excellent at excreting water, as any beer-drinker knows, but they are not well adapted to excreting sodium because our evolutionary ancestors had little access to sodium. There weren't any salt shakers in their caves and no salt licks out on the plain!

### BEANO

Many times, when I advise patients to follow a low-fat diet and to eat more plants and fewer animals, they return to my office praising the diet for its good effect on their weight, diabetes, high blood pressure, and gout, but they complain that they have "gas"—they are passing more gas. The reason this occurs is that many vegetables—especially beans, broccoli, cabbage, and cauliflower—contain non-absorbable oligosaccharides. These oligosaccharides consist of chains of simple sugars (glucose, galactose, fructose) linked together with alpha bonds. The human intestine cannot absorb oligosaccharides directly, because it lacks the enzyme needed to break alpha bonds.

That means that the oligosaccharides are not absorbed in the small intestine; they continue on to the colon where they are metabolized by bacteria blessed with the necessary alpha-breaking enzymes. Bacteria are messy eaters; they produce acid and gas, as every vegetarian knows.

That's where Beano fits in. Beano (a product of KPharma, Inc.) is *alpha-galactosidase,* the enzyme we need to break up oligosaccharides and absorb them. Beano is available in most pharmacies and grocery stores. People put a few drops of Beano on their first bite of beans or cauliflower, and they can eat the rest of their meal without the worry of gas. Beano is purified from a common bread mold, so people with severe mold allergy should not use the product. But Beano is a help for the rest of us.

## Dietary Beliefs, Myths, and Fads

With regard to eating meat, there are two extremes of opinion: those who advocate eating a vegetarian, low-protein, high-carbohydrate diet, and those who advocate a high-protein—therefore high-meat—diet. The former group is represented by Nathan Pritikin,[7] myself, and three billion people outside of the United States and Europe. The latter group is represented by Robert Atkins[8] and Michael and Mary Eades.[9]

The fundamental premise of the high-protein diet is that it reduces weight and promotes good health by reducing the release of insulin from the pancreas. When food arrives in the stomach, the hormone insulin is released from the pancreas. Carbohydrates are especially potent stimulators of insulin release. Insulin acts on many organs in the body, driving blood glucose (sugar) into cells, storing the glucose in various storage forms, and building up muscles and other tissues. Dr. Eades's contention is that this process of building up tissues counteracts the desired effect of losing weight and contributes to coronary artery disease. The high-protein advocate also hopes that by reducing the demand for insulin from the pancreas, development of diabetes can be delayed or avoided.

It's all nonsense. Almost all natural high-protein foods are high-fat foods. I asked the "Diet Balancer"[10] program on my computer to search for high-protein, low-fat foods, and it located only four items, including tuna fish! Any high-protein diet using natural foods is automatically a high-fat diet. And where do you think all that fat in the diet leads? Recall that fats have 9 calories per gram, while carbohydrates have 4.

There is a more insidious danger in the high-protein strategy. Protein contains nitrogen, unlike carbohydrates and fat. Most of the protein consumed in high-protein diets is burned, releasing nitrogen that must be excreted by the kidneys. Dr. Eades recommends consuming 80 (if one is sedentary) to 144 (for athletes) grams of protein a day. The human body can only incorporate 30 grams of dietary protein into muscle each day, assuming vigorous exercise. The remaining protein is simply burned, releasing nitrogen, which damages the kidneys.

People are born with four times as much kidney function as they actually need. That is the reserve capacity that protects people from kidney failure in the event of loss or damage to the kidneys. In civilized Western countries, kidney function declines steadily with age, so that by the age of eighty a person has lost nearly 50 percent of the kidney capacity that was present at age twenty. In agrarian societies, where people eat a high-carbohydrate diet, this steep decline in kidney function does not occur. It has not been proven that the decline in kidney function in Western societies occurs because of the overconsumption of protein, but it is the chief suspect.[11]

## Fiber

Dietitians and physicians recommend adding more fiber to the diet. *Fiber* is the term for the part of food that is not absorbed and ends up in the stool. At first thought, you might wonder why anyone would encourage you to put things in your diet that aren't absorbed, but there are good reasons for doing so. Fiber in the diet increases the transit time through the intestine so that fats are less well absorbed. This helps with weight loss. And fiber prevents the dieter from becoming constipated—an especially important consideration when taking phen-Prozac. To judge from the ads on television during the nightly news, "irregularity" is about the worst calamity that can befall a person, causing loss of job and family and causing one's body to be distorted by wavy lines on the TV screen.

Fiber comes in two types: soluble and insoluble. You should get some of both types in your diet. Soluble fibers are those found in apples, oatmeal, and Metamucil, for example. They are called "soluble" because they dissolve in water. Soluble fiber is helpful in lowering blood cholesterol level and it helps prevent heart attacks, as any box of Quaker Oats will tell you.

Insoluble fiber is not soluble in water. These high-molecular-weight fibers have less effect on cholesterol level, but epidemiological studies suggest that insoluble fiber is helpful in preventing colon cancer. Colon cancer—the number two killer in the United States—is virtually unheard of in vegetarian societies. Moreover, fiber of this type is useful in lowering colonic pressure so people are less likely to develop diverticulosis. Diverticulosis, common in Americans over age fifty, is the formation of pouches branching off from the colon. The pouches can become plugged and infected, or they may bleed.

**Fiber Sources**

| Source | Portion | Approximate Grams Fiber* |
|---|---|---|
| Apple | Small | 2.8 |
| Banana | Medium | 2.0 |
| Beans (kidney) | 1/2 cup | 5.5 |
| Beans (lima) | 1/2 cup | 4.4 |
| Bread (whole wheat) | Slice | 2.0 |
| Broccoli | 3/4 cup | 5.0 |
| Carrots (raw) | 4 sticks | 1.7 |
| Green Beans | 1/2 cup | 2.1 |
| Green Peas (canned) | 1/2 cup | 3.0 |
| Oat Bran | 1/2 cup | 3.0 |
| Orange | Small | 3.0 |
| Peach | Medium | 2.0 |
| Pear | Small | 3.0 |
| Potato | Small | 4.2 |
| Rice (brown) | 1/2 cup | 5.5 |
| Watermelon | Thick slice | 2.8 |

*Fiber values are approximate and may vary.

FIGURE 8.1

Diverticulosis is rare in the Third World, where diets are high in insoluble fiber.

## Fad Diets

Many times, patients have brought me books on their favorite fad diet: high-protein, low-fat, high-vitamin, low-yeast, you name it. They asked my opinion. I usually pooh-poohed the diets, insisting that a balanced diet was best. Moderation was my watchword. The usual sequel to this story was that the patient took the book home, followed the diet, and returned to my office boasting about how much weight they had lost in three weeks. I usually handed them another "pooh-pooh platter."

The fact is that any diet that restricts food choices will generate some weight loss in the short run. A Kosher diet will work, an all-chicken diet will work, even a diet restricted to yellow foods will work—in the short run. Any program like this works in the short run because the need to follow a rule in food selection keeps the obese patient's mind on the obesity, and the limited availability of Kosher, chicken, or yellow foods prevents the patient from eating other fattening foods they would otherwise eat.

The real test of diets is this: what is the patient's weight in six months? Not many of the people who brought me the books even remembered what the book was about when they weighed in at my office six months later and discovered that they had gained back all their weight.

*The real test of diets is this: what is the patient's weight in six months?*

## Yo-Yo Dieting

There has been a lot of concern about yo-yo dieting. Yo-yo dieting refers to repeatedly losing and regaining weight. Two problems have been alleged. First, an epidemiological study suggested that yo-yo dieters had a higher rate of death and heart attacks than obese people who stayed at a constant weight, even if both had the same average weight. Subsequent, more careful studies showed that this allegation was untrue. Moral: never believe the first study.

The second charge was that yo-yo dieting conditioned the body to hold on to excess weight by lowering a person's basal metabolic rate, making the body hold onto calories more efficiently. This charge is marginally true at best. The maximum spread of basal metabolic rates is only about 15 percent, yo-yo dieting or not. When one looks at yo-yo dieters specifically, one is looking at a population of patients with poor appetite and impulse control. The fact that they also have poor weight control does not establish a causal relationship between yo-yo dieting and metabolism.

It is dangerous to teach yo-yo dieters that they are doomed to failure. They will assume that their metabolism is so depressed that they cannot lose weight, and they may give up in despair. With the information outlined in this book, there is no need for despair.

CHAPTER NINE

# What Exercise Does and Doesn't Do

Whether you use phen-Prozac to lose weight or you diet voluntarily to lose weight, the following is still true:

calories in – calories out = change in weight

You can't beat thermodynamics.[1] We are what we eat—or, to put it more accurately, we are what we eat minus what we do.

Everyone who wants to lose weight should try exercising on an exercycle with an ergonometer that reads out the number of calories burned in a given period of exercise. I have to cycle twenty minutes to burn off the equivalent of one beer. Fat is a very efficient storage form for energy—that is why the body bothers to make the stuff!

A single pound of fat contains 3,600 calories[2] of potential energy. My five hundred phen-Prozac patients lost 8,000 pounds of fat in a year and a half. There was enough energy in that fat to boil 17,000 gallons of water, generate 4,000 kilowatt-hours of electricity, or power the Space Shuttle for 2,000 feet after lift-off!

You might think you would have to exercise a lot to lose even a little weight, and you would be right. A little attention to diet combined with the use of medications to lower hunger is undoubtedly an easier route.

Look at the numbers. The rate at which a young man burns calories while engaging in various activities is shown in the following table:

| Activity | Calories Burned per Hour |
|---|---|
| clerical work | 115 |
| walking at 3 mph | 240 |
| riding bicycle at 13 mph | 480 |
| exercising on stairclimber | 660 |
| jogging at 7 mph | 840 |

The increase in the rate at which calories are burned while jogging as compared to sitting at a desk is impressive, but let's look at the situation realistically. The young man is not going to jog twenty-four hours a day. He might jog for one hour a day—or, more likely, half an hour. In that half hour, he will burn off 420 calories. In the remaining twenty-three hours of sedentary activity, he burns off 23 × 115, or 2,645 calories, for a total of 2,645 + 420, or 3,065 calories.

Compare that figure to the same young man sitting at a desk all day, doing no exercise. He burns off 24 × 115, or 2,760 calories. On days when he runs for half an hour, he burns off only 11 percent more calories than on days when he only works at a desk. He would need to jog half an hour every day for twelve days to lose a pound of fat![3]

The number of calories that the young man would have burned off by jogging for half an hour—420 calories—is the equivalent of one Big Mac (530 calories) or one bag of french fries (400 calories). If the young man had simply left one food item off his lunch tray, he could have skipped jogging for the day and his caloric balance would have been the same!

And, aerobic exercise increases the levels of neuropeptide Y in the appestat, meaning, exercise increases hunger. If an athlete eats to the point where the extra hunger is satisfied, the athlete will have taken in enough extra calories to match the calories burned in the exercise.[4]

## Why Exercise Is Good

You might think, after all that, I would recommend that dieters give up on exercise. Far from it! I do recommend exercise: aerobic exercise. All of my phen-Prozac patients who were successful in losing weight were committed to a daily exercise routine. But, as we have seen, the effectiveness of the routine cannot be explained solely on the basis of calorie computations. There must have been a psychological effect from the exercise that helped to keep patients on the diet plan. The exercise served as a reminder not to eat an extra sandwich. It improved their sense of well-being and gave them a positive self-image. Being successful with the exercise program, they expected to be successful on the diet, and they were!

Exercise confers health benefits that are not related to body weight. Exercise increases the muscle mass of the body, enabling it to burn off unwanted calories faster. Aerobic exercise improves the aerobic capacity of the heart and raises levels of HDL, the good component of cholesterol that prevents heart attack by removing lipids from the walls of the arteries.

---

*All of my phen-Prozac patients who were successful losing weight were committed to a daily exercise routine.*

---

I believe that the SSRIs have a direct effect in enabling my patients to adhere to their exercise programs. Patients taking phen-Prozac are much more likely to exercise than patients who take phentermine alone, even at early stages in the medical program before a difference in weight loss is apparent. SSRIs are known to have the effect of reducing mood swings. I think the same effect helps the dieter stick to an exercise routine.

## How to Exercise Safely

Exercise, for obese people, should be undertaken carefully. Obese patients with known or possible heart disease should consult their physician before starting to exercise. Details of the exercise plan should be discussed thoroughly.

Patients should vary both the type and amount of exercise they do each day. Tired, sore muscles that have sustained cellular injury need forty-eight hours to heal. If the dieter insists on exercising sore muscles on successive days, tissue damage accumulates until there is a breakdown. Therefore, exercises must be varied. If the dieter proposes to work out on successive days, exercises should be arranged in alternating "upper body" and "lower body" days. People should never "exercise through pain." Pain has a purpose: to prevent further tissue injury. Don't ignore the signal.

Dieters should always do stretches and warm-up exercises before getting to the "real" exercise. Don't be too eager to get to the barbells or start the clock on a four-mile run. Warm up first or you may wind up in your doctor's office with torn ligaments and strained muscles.

Obese people should not attempt to run at the same speed or exercise as long as thinner people who are in better condition. Pulling the heavier body weight, an obese person does not need to run as far or as quickly to burn off the same number of calories as a thinner athlete does. The obese athlete has a pair of barbells built in. See Figure 9.1.

There is more information in this figure than I need to make my point, but seeing the calorie consumption from several forms of exercise is helpful. The point is, a 210-pound person can burn off as many calories by walking at a rate of four miles per hour as a 110-pound person can burn off by running, with less risk to the knees and ankles.

## Walking

Walking is great exercise. Just don't stop to chat with the neighbors. If you have thirty minutes to walk, spend fifteen minutes

Approximate Energy Expenditure in Selected Activities for People of Different Weights (Calories per 30 Minutes)*

| Activity | Weight (Pounds) | | | | | |
|---|---|---|---|---|---|---|
| | 110 | 130 | 150 | 170 | 190 | 210 |
| Aerobic dancing | | | | | | |
| "walking pace" | 99 | 114 | 132 | 150 | 168 | 186 |
| "jogging pace" | 159 | 186 | 213 | 243 | 270 | 300 |
| "running pace" | 204 | 240 | 276 | 315 | 351 | 387 |
| Basketball | 207 | 243 | 282 | 318 | 357 | 396 |
| Canoeing–leisure | 66 | 78 | 90 | 102 | 114 | 126 |
| Canoeing–racing | 156 | 183 | 210 | 237 | 267 | 294 |
| Carpentry | 78 | 93 | 105 | 120 | 135 | 147 |
| Cycling–5.5 mph | 96 | 114 | 132 | 147 | 165 | 183 |
| Cycling–9.4 mph | 150 | 177 | 204 | 231 | 258 | 285 |
| Dancing–ballroom | 78 | 90 | 105 | 117 | 132 | 144 |
| Dancing–disco | 156 | 183 | 210 | 237 | 267 | 294 |
| Gardening | 150 | 177 | 204 | 231 | 258 | 285 |
| Golf | 129 | 150 | 174 | 195 | 219 | 243 |
| Judo | 294 | 345 | 399 | 450 | 504 | 558 |
| Lying or sitting down | 33 | 39 | 45 | 51 | 57 | 63 |
| Mopping floor | 96 | 105 | 120 | 138 | 153 | 171 |
| Running | | | | | | |
| 11.5 minutes per mile | 204 | 240 | 276 | 315 | 351 | 387 |
| 9 minutes per mile | 291 | 342 | 393 | 447 | 498 | 552 |
| 7 minutes per mile | 366 | 417 | 468 | 522 | 573 | 624 |
| 5.5 minutes per mile | 435 | 513 | 591 | 669 | 747 | 828 |
| Skiing, cross-country | 216 | 252 | 291 | 330 | 369 | 408 |
| Standing quietly | 39 | 45 | 51 | 57 | 66 | 72 |
| Swimming | | | | | | |
| backstroke | 255 | 300 | 345 | 390 | 435 | 486 |
| crawl | 192 | 228 | 261 | 297 | 330 | 366 |
| Table tennis | 102 | 120 | 138 | 156 | 174 | 195 |
| Tennis | 165 | 192 | 222 | 252 | 282 | 312 |
| Walking | | | | | | |
| 3 mph | 102 | 114 | 126 | 138 | 153 | 165 |
| 4 mph | 120 | 141 | 162 | 186 | 207 | 228 |

*Adapted from *The High Energy Factor,* by Bernard Gutin. Copyright © 1983 by Bernard Gutin and Gail Kessler. Reprinted by permission of Random House, Inc.

FIGURE 9.1

walking out and fifteen minutes walking back. Move quickly and continuously and swing your arms. If you walk the dog, have him do his business before he walks with you. Better yet, leave the dog at home.

Walk on a good surface, in good shoes. The shoes should be soft with good heel and arch supports. If the shoes hurt, purchase new ones.

The best surface is, not surprisingly, the track at the local school. Tracks are built the way they are precisely so they will not cause foot problems. The next best surface is dry, level grass or a black asphalt road surface. Do not walk for long periods of time on concrete or wood; these surfaces are too hard and can cause heel spurs *(plantar fasciitis).*

## Jogging

It is especially important for joggers to stretch out their Achilles tendons before exercise and also before bed. Joggers should stand with their hands on the wall and walk backward, keeping their heels on the floor, and rock forward to stretch the Achilles tendon. Not only does this simple exercise prevent ankle sprains, it prevents nocturnal calf cramps as well.

Joggers and walkers should drink plenty of water during hot weather, and they should wear sunscreen appropriately to avoid sunburn.

It is perfectly acceptable to jog slowly. In fact it is preferable to do so, if you are heavy, to protect the knees and feet. There is a married couple in my neighborhood who goes around the block every day, the wife walking and the husband jogging, side by side. That's fine.

No one expects the overweight jogger to work up to run the marathon or a four-minute mile. The purpose of the exercise is to get healthy, so it behooves the jogger to exercise in a healthful way. The goal is to exercise consistently.

Maintain a pace in running where you feel you are getting the benefits of the exercise without being overly challenged. Exercise is aerobic (good for you) as long as you can keep up a conversation while you are at it. It is not important to actually talk, only that you could talk if you wanted to. If you are so breathless that you would not be able to talk, the exercise has become anaerobic (bad for you); in this case, slow the pace or stop to rest.

### Weight Lifting

If you feel compelled to lift weights as a form of exercise because of adolescent fantasies about big biceps, please please please lift only light weights using many repetitions, rather than heavy weights with a few "reps." Move quickly from one exercise to another. You are far less likely to get hurt this way, and you will actually improve your health rather than injure it.

---

*Phen-Prozac therapy can take pounds off, but where they come off is determined largely by genetics.*

---

There is a tendency for novice weight lifters to take a cue from the Arnold Schwarzenegger types in the gym, who lift heavy weights with a few reps, taking a long time between sets. You figure that if Arnie looks so good, his way must be the right way. But don't be fooled. Lifting big weights can build bulky muscles, but the muscle built in this way has low aerobic capacity, and lifting heavy weights does nothing for your blood pressure or HDL level. Olympic weight lifters don't live long. On the other hand, lighter weights and lots of reps done quickly build muscles with greater aerobic capacity, improve HDL levels, lower blood pressure, and extend life.

## Patterns of Weight Loss

There are different kinds of fat in the human body. The fat around the intestine and on the back of the neck are the most metabolically active, meaning the fat in these areas is broken down and removed in response to diet more easily than fat elsewhere in the body. The fat around hips and thighs is much less active (and more difficult to get rid of). Fat in the breasts is moderately active.

When women lose weight, it tends to come off the belly first, breasts second, hips and thighs last. There is some variability, but our basic body shape is inherited: we look like our parents. And we lose weight in the same way as they do. Phen-Prozac therapy can take pounds off, but where they come off is determined largely by genetics.

You can change the pattern of weight loss only to a limited degree with exercise. If you exercise your legs you can add muscle and paradoxically increase the diameter of your thighs, but fat will still come off your belly and breasts first. Over time, however, your legs will also become trimmer.

## Use Your Big Muscles

Many people love to exercise, and many despise it. Forty percent of American men exercise regularly. They are the ones for whom Sports Authority and Athletic Express stores were built. They are the ones for whom 1,001 varieties of cross-training shoes exist. The remaining 60 percent of men, however, are sedentary. Most women get some daily exercise—they have that much self-esteem—but no creature on earth is as passive as the sedentary American male. Only Jabba the Hut could compare.

Exercise expert Covert Bailey, in his amusing and informative *Fit or Fat* series of books and videotapes, addresses the question, "How should a person exercise who needs to lose weight but hates to exercise?" What is the most efficient form of exercise for people who don't want to spend a lot of time exercising?

The answer is to use the largest muscles in the body: the leg muscles. The best exercises for these muscles are running, bicycling, or—Bailey's favorite—the alpine ski machine. The stairclimber is also good, as is the treadmill.

But not the rowing machine. The rowing machine is dangerous for out-of-shape people. I have seen too many back injuries from it. You could learn to use the thing safely, with proper instruction, but there are so many better toys to play with.

You can lose weight by swimming or playing racquetball, but you have to exercise much longer in these sports because they use smaller muscles. Tennis is good exercise if you are a good tennis player. But if you can't keep up a volley, forget tennis—or take lessons.

Housework counts as exercise, if done vigorously and continuously. Going up and down stairs with a basket of laundry does wonders for the legs and thighs. Sex can count as exercise, too, for anyone who can last long enough to get the heart rate up. According to one study, having sex burns 100 to 150 calories—nearly equal to the amount of calories burned in a twenty-minute walk.[5]

## Spare Those Knees

Morbidly obese people should not do any exercise that involves bouncing on their knees and ankles, such as jumping jacks or volleyball. Bouncing on these joints can cause or exacerbate osteoarthritis, and can cause acute rupture of supporting tendons and ligaments. Fast walking burns calories just as effectively as slow jogging does, and it puts less strain on the knees. There is always one foot on the ground when one is walking. When running, both feet are off the ground during part of each cycle. When the leading foot lands on the ground, it comes down with a force equal to seven times the runner's body weight. No wonder so many injuries occur! In the beginning, obese people should focus on fast walking rather than jogging.

An even safer way is to exercise in water. The buoyancy takes most of the weight off the knees, and the resistance of the water adds to the effectiveness of the exercise. Swimming is not the most efficient way to use the pool, however, because swimming uses mainly arm motion. A better way to exercise in the pool is to walk forcefully through the water—essentially, jog in the water—making use of the powerful leg muscles. Many obese people would be embarrassed to be seen jogging in the water, or fear they might get in the way of swimmers, but many community pools have scheduled times reserved for aerobic exercise in the pool. Call your local pool to find out.

## Have Fun

The most important piece of advice I have regarding exercise is this: have fun. You will not keep up the exercise if you don't enjoy it. One of my patients got her exercise by square dancing daily. She loved it! It is always better to exercise with company, and friends are more motivating than strangers.

If you are exercising when no one else is home, turn on the TV or listen to the radio. You're more likely to exercise longer if you watch Maury Povich than if you watch the clock.

## Keep Moving

The calories you burn off at the gym are a small fraction of the total that you burn off during the rest of the day. Live so that you are using energy all day long. I have noticed that chronically obese patients tend to sit very still. Whether they are listening to me or waiting in the waiting room, they are motionless. Chronically thin patients are constantly moving, squirming, changing magazines, correcting their children. Obese people are like the angelfish in my aquarium; thin people are like the guppies.

I have seen this phenomenon when I visit my daughter's school. I peek in the windows in different classrooms, and I notice that the overweight teachers are sitting at their desks talking to the children. The thin teachers are pacing at the blackboard or walking up and down aisles.

---

*Live so that you are using energy all day long.*

---

These are generalizations, of course; not all obese people sit motionless and not all thin people pace. But if you notice that you tend to be a still person, you are not helping yourself lose weight. Cultivate mobility. Get rid of your chair. If you drive to work, don't park near the entrance. Get out and walk; enjoy the sunshine. Take the stairs instead of the elevator. A person who follows this advice may not need to depend on the gym or labor so long on the treadmill.

CHAPTER TEN

# Obesity-Related Problems

Let's take a close look at some facts and issues related to obesity.

## Diabetes

One major way that obesity endangers the health of Americans is by causing diabetes. Diabetes mellitus[1] is a disease in which blood glucose (sugar) is elevated above normal levels. A high blood sugar level damages the walls of blood vessels and leads to a host of problems involving the eyes, nerves, and kidneys. Diabetes also accelerates the process of atherosclerosis, leading to heart attacks and strokes. Seven million people in America have diabetes, most of them obese. Of every four people with diabetes, only three have been diagnosed.

There are two types of diabetes. Physicians have cycled through a number of naming systems but have settled on *Type I* and *Type II.* Twenty percent of diabetic patients have Type I diabetes. These patients tend to be younger, thinner, and sicker than Type II patients. Type I patients take insulin shots to stay alive, because the pancreas has lost its capacity to produce insulin.

Insulin is the hormone that tells the muscles how much glucose to take in from the bloodstream. The job of insulin is to assure that the brain always has a ready supply of glucose, the fuel on which the brain is totally dependent. Muscles can use other metabolic fuels if the glucose supply is low. If the muscles could extract glucose from the bloodstream at will, the blood glucose level would fall during exercise and brain function would shut down. So glucose is required to have a ticket—insulin—to get into the muscle cells, to ensure that the brain gets its share of glucose. Glucose doesn't need a ticket to get into the brain.

The pancreas puts out a constant low level of insulin to take care of the glucose that constantly percolates out of the liver, and it puts out a surge of insulin whenever it senses the arrival of food in the stomach, to handle the large amount of dietary glucose coming in.

You can understand why the blood glucose level goes up in Type I diabetics, who cannot produce insulin to regulate glucose levels, and why taking insulin shots largely corrects the problem.

But what about Type II diabetics? They produce normal or greater-than-normal levels of insulin. Why do they have a problem?

Type II diabetics are resistant to insulin. The insulin in their bodies does not work as well on muscles to induce them to extract glucose from the bloodstream. As a result, glucose hangs around in the arteries and causes damage. The tendency to be resistant to insulin is a consequence of genetics, age, and obesity.[2] If your family has a history of diabetes, you are likely to become diabetic if you get old enough and heavy enough. If your family has no history of diabetes, you are unlikely to become diabetic no matter how old or heavy you become.

Avoiding obesity while you are young will make you less likely to become diabetic later. If you are a Type II diabetic and lose weight, the diabetes will probably go away. Many of my patients who had Type II diabetes before they went on phen-Prozac are no longer diabetic after losing weight on the program.

---

*Many of my patients who had Type II diabetes before they went on phen-Prozac are no longer diabetic after losing weight on the program.*

---

If a Type II diabetic has diabetes for too long without relief, the pancreas gets tired and loses its ability to produce insulin. The Type II diabetic must then be placed on insulin shots to preserve life. For these diabetics, it is too late for phen-Prozac to cure the diabetes. Nevertheless, it is important to reduce obesity so the dose of insulin can be minimized and the diabetes will be easier to control.

## The Diabetic Diet

Many patients, when they learn they have diabetes, assume that all they have to do to control it is reduce the amount of sugar in their diets. Alas, it is not so simple. The body is perfectly capable of converting fat into sugar, sugar into fat, fat into protein, protein into sugar, and so on. The important thing to watch in the diabetic diet is not sugar but calories.

Each unit of fat ingested can effectively generate two units of sugar. The diabetic really needs a low-fat diet, not a low-sugar diet. A piece of melon contains as much sugar as a piece of pie, but a diabetic is better off eating the melon because the pie has a stick of margarine in it.

Diabetics often go wild consuming sweeteners such as saccharin and aspartame. This may not be a problem, although I personally dislike the taste of artificial sweeteners. There was some question about the possibility that saccharin causes bladder cancer, and aspartame causes headaches in many people. A teaspoonful of sugar doesn't have a lot of calories; I would rather see diabetics and obese people drinking a regular Coke instead of a Diet Coke, if only they could forego the cheeseburger and fries that often go with it. There are tremendously more calories in a bag of french fries than in a regular Coke.

## Precose Precautions

*Precose* is a new medicine for obese Type II diabetics. I don't have a very high opinion of it. It's like "reverse Beano," inhibiting the enzymes that break down complex carbohydrates in the gut for absorption. Unabsorbed carbohydrates pass on through the large intestine where colonic bacteria get hold of them, ferment them, and turn them into acid and gas. If Beano was designed to prevent gas, what do you think Precose does?

Pharmaceutical companies, physicians, and obese patients should shift their focus away from inhibiting absorption of food. There are better solutions to obesity, and to spend so much time and money to block absorption of excess food in rich Americans, when so many in the world are hungry, seems like a backward approach to solving these problems.

## Sleep Apnea

Sleep apnea is a common, dangerous disease often not recognized by the patient or the doctor. Of every four people in America with this disorder, three have not been diagnosed. Almost all sleep apnea patients are obese. In these patients, the walls of the throat close up during sleep and breathing is obstructed for a minute or more. During that period, the patient's chest is moving, trying to expel or suck in air, but no air is moving. Sounds bad, and it is! The oxygen concentration in the blood falls precipitously and the carbon dioxide level rises.

When the carbon dioxide level rises high enough, the patient is awakened just enough to recover the muscle tone in the throat, temporarily relieving the obstruction. The patient's sleeping partner can often make the diagnosis. All patients with sleep apnea snore, although the majority of people who snore do not have sleep apnea. When loud snoring is interrupted by periods of silence, during which the chest is moving up and down but no air is flowing at the nose or mouth, the patient can be recognized to have sleep apnea. The more definitive, expensive way to make the diagnosis is for the patient to undergo a polysomnogram—a sleep study performed in a sleep laboratory.

Patients who have sleep apnea are drowsy during the day. They often get into automobile wrecks because they fall asleep at the wheel. Their work quality suffers. Many patients drink caffeine or pop "uppers" to keep themselves awake during the day, then take sleeping pills at night, which is dangerous. Smoking and alcohol make sleep apnea worse. Untreated sleep apnea can lead to enlargement of the heart and heart failure. Patients may die suddenly in their sleep from cardiac arrhythmia induced by low blood oxygen.

The condition can be immediately corrected in most patients by using continuous positive airway pressure (CPAP). The patient wears a little mask over the nose at night, instilling a thin stream of air into the nostrils to keep the airway open. I am not sure why this technique works, but I am glad it does because the old treatment for sleep apnea was a tracheostomy!

CPAP does not solve the primary problem, but it can protect the patient from the worst consequences of the disease and allow time to look for a more permanent answer. Some patients make immediate inroads into the disease by stopping smoking or excessive drinking. Others can be helped by a tonsillectomy or an operation called a pharyngoplasty, in which excess tissue in the back of the throat is carved away.

But the high road to a cure is to lose weight, and there is no better, faster, or more reliable way to do that than with phen-Prozac. I have many patients whose sleep apnea has been permanently cured by weight loss.

## Gallstones

Gallstones are stones, ranging in size from a BB to a golf ball, that form in the gallbladder of some people. Because the stones are formed from cholesterol, you might think they would be most common in people with high blood cholesterol, but such is not the case. The population most at risk for gallstones is obese people generally, whether they have high cholesterol or not.

Existing gallstones grow the fastest; new gallstones are formed most readily in obese patients who are losing weight on a diet. This is not an argument against dieting. The great majority of obese individuals who form a gallstone while dieting would have formed the gallstone eventually.

*The population most at risk for gallstones is obese people, whether they have high cholesterol or not.*

Gallstones can obstruct the outlet of the gallbladder, causing severe pain and nausea. Once a patient develops a gallstone, the usual treatment is to remove the gallbladder surgically. Cholecystectomy—surgery to remove the gallbladder—has recently become an easier proposition. In most cases, the gallbladder can be removed through a special tube, called a laparoscope, that is inserted through a small incision in the navel. No longer do patients wind up with long, jagged scars on their abdomen. Cholecystectomy is the second most common surgery performed in the United States, after the appendectomy. One adult in twelve gets a cholecystectomy.

There is a medicine called Actigall that dissolves gallstones, but it takes six months to work and the success rate is 50 percent. Surgery is generally better.

## Wrinkles

Many obese patients are concerned that when they lose weight they will be left with unsightly loose folds of skin. It's a legitimate concern. If the obesity was severe and much weight is lost, the patient is left with folds of skin hanging down. The situation is worse under the following conditions:

- The patient is elderly or has had severe sun exposure. In either case, the skin is less elastic.
- The patient has lost or never had normal muscle mass.
- The patient is genetically prone to wrinkling.

To some extent, the skin tightens up with time. Patients should not rush to a plastic surgeon immediately after reaching their goal weight. But if there are still bags and folds in the skin after six months, patients may consult a plastic surgeon. There are many excellent techniques whereby the excess skin can be removed. These techniques have been around for years, but the wonderful thing is that now, thanks to phen-Prozac, neither the surgeon nor the patient has to worry that the obesity will return to restretch the skin.

## Surgical Approaches to Obesity

There are several surgical methods for treating obesity, among them gastric stapling, liposuction, and "tummy tucks."

### Gastric Stapling

Of the many surgical approaches to treating obesity, only gastric stapling is still used with any frequency. The idea behind gastric stapling is to reduce weight by causing the patient to feel more full at an early stage of each meal. Readers of this book will appreciate that the procedure does not obviously reduce the production of leptin nor directly act on the appestat. You would think that the patients would be terribly hungry all the time and, like Tantalus in the Greek myth, would be unable to satisfy their hunger by eating, given the small size of the new stomach. However, patients do not appear to be as hungry as one might expect.

In gastric stapling, the stomach is cut into two parts (see Figure 10.1). The open ends of the cut stomach are stapled shut, creating a new, smaller stomach still attached to the esophagus. The small intestine is cut through, and the end connected to the rest of the intestine is brought up and attached to the new small stomach.

If this seems like major surgery to you, it certainly is! And keep in mind that this surgery is performed on obese patients who are not in great shape to begin with. There is a high rate of complications, including tearing apart of the staple line

**Gastric Stapling**

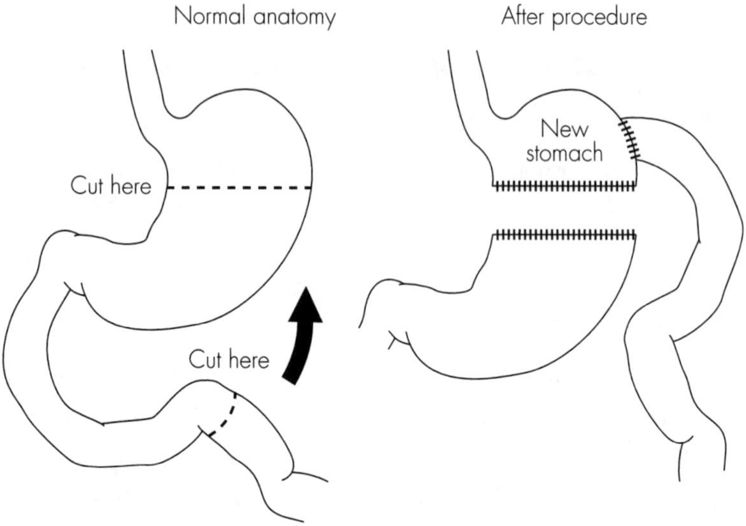


FIGURE 10.1

on the stomach and tearing apart of the incision line on the skin. The former problem requires an immediate second surgery. There is a higher-than-average frequency of heart attacks and strokes in older obese patients as a result of gastric stapling, and obese surgical patients are prone to pneumonia and blood clots.

After gastric stapling, all patients lose weight at first, but many experience side effects. There is a tendency for heartburn because the reduced size of the stomach puts pressure on food and acid to travel back up into the esophagus. Because the normal pylorus—the valve between the normal stomach and the small intestine—is no longer part of the circuit, food is dumped into the intestine at an uncontrolled rate. This may lead to diarrhea and bloating. Bile can leak upward into the stomach or the esophagus. Scarring can close off the bile duct, the stomach, or the intestine. However, such serious postsurgical complications are rare.

More common is the formation of peptic ulcers at the site of stapling, either in the new stomach or in the pouch from the old stomach. To avoid this problem, patients must take medicines to reduce the acid content of the stomach.

Gastric stapling should be thought of as an absolute last resort for overweight people, given its high rate of complications.

## Liposuction

Liposuction is a procedure in which small incisions are made in the skin and fat is literally sucked out of the body with a vacuum-cleaner-like device. The advantage of this procedure is that excess fat is removed from specific parts of the body. As discussed in Chapter 9, phen-Prozac can remove fat from the body generally, but it cannot control which parts of the body are trimmed. Overweight patients who are dissatisfied with the diameter of their hips and thighs may be tempted to resort to liposuction to remove fat from those specific areas.

Buyer beware! While patients look great shortly after liposuction, the reduction in fat mass leads to decreased levels of leptin since there are fewer fat cells to secrete it. Consequently, there is increased hunger and more eating. The suction process never removes all the fat cells from any area. Some fat is left behind for technical and cosmetic reasons. The fat cells that are left inevitably enlarge, leaving the patient with a lumpy, bumpy appearance, like a pillowcase stuffed with toys. Adding to that problem are the scars left from the incisions through which the liposuction apparatus was inserted. I have not seen any liposuction patients who were happy with the result a year after the procedure.

*I have not seen any liposuction patients who were happy with the result a year after the procedure.*

**Tummy Tucks**

Some of my patients who lost a hundred pounds or more were left with bags of stretched out, excess skin hanging down from their abdomens. Not all. In many of the patients, the skin contracted as the patient did. There seems to be a genetic difference among people in this regard.

While I discourage liposuction, I have seen good results from abdomenoplasty, surgery in which rolls of excess skin are removed. The scar that is left is similar to a C-section scar; tucked away in the pubic hair, it's almost invisible. Excess skin elsewhere, left over after weight loss, can be removed by various means.

For best results, patients should defer surgery until they have lost all their excess weight or reached a stable level of weight. If surgery is done too soon, further loss of weight could result in new folds of skin. If the weight is not stable, weight regained could threaten the cosmetic results.

CHAPTER ELEVEN

# Myths About Obesity

I hear the following complaint often:

> Jane: "Doctor, the reason I can't lose weight is that my metabolism is too slow. My husband, David, can eat anything he wants and he stays skinny. If I even look at chocolate, I put on weight."

This statement is interesting for several reasons. First, Jane (and most other people) believe that there is a wide range of metabolic rates among individuals. Jane believes that she is cursed with a low metabolic rate while her husband is blessed with a fast one. This may be true, but it is unlikely to be true to the degree that Jane imagines.

The total metabolic rate is equal to the sum of the basal metabolic rate (BMR) plus the extra metabolism generated by exercise. The BMR does vary among individuals. If you take into account age, gender, and body surface area, there is a 15-percent variation in BMR among individuals—but the variation is *only* 15 percent, not enough to account for the wide variation in body sizes.

Some studies have shown that obese people are less active than their thinner counterparts, but Figure 9.1 (page 156) shows that heavier people burn off more calories in exercise because they are pulling greater body weight. Even if Jane moves less often and less briskly than her husband, her energy consumption might not be much lower than his.

Second, Jane's perception is that David eats more than she does. This may or may not be true. Numerous studies have examined the reliability of dietary data voluntarily reported by individuals. The studies are consistent in showing that obese people underreport their consumption by 40 percent, compared with 15 percent among normal-weight controls. A graph showing the distribution of food consumption among obese and non-obese individuals shows two overlapping bell-shaped curves (Figure 11.1). There are some thin people who eat more than some overweight people, to be sure, but not many. There are many more overweight people who eat more than normal-weight people.

Third, Jane's choice of words shows a fundamental difference in thinking, compared to her spouse. In just three sentences, she mentions twice that she is thinking about food during the day. She says, "David can eat anything he wants." Probably David does not even think about what he wants to eat until he looks at a menu. Thinking about food is not one of his hobbies. Jane complains, "If I even look at chocolate . . ." and

**Amount of Food Consumed by Obese and Non-Obese People**

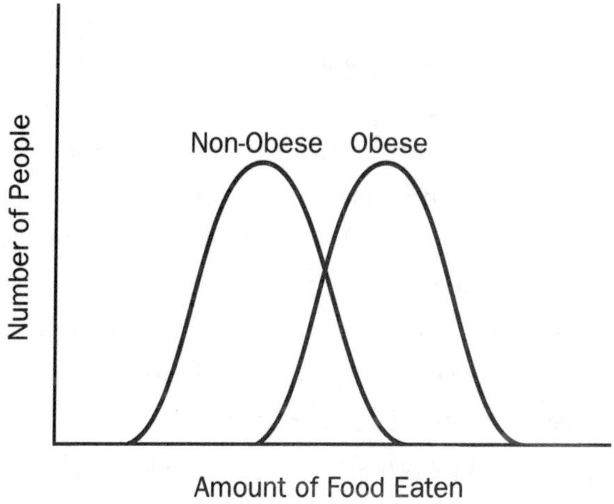


FIGURE 11.1

so on. I suspect that Jane knows exactly where the chocolate is in her house, and David doesn't. The reason for the difference between them is not that Jane is depraved, it is that Jane is so frequently hungry. Set David on a raft in the ocean for a few days, deprive him of food, and you'll see: when he returns home, he'll pay close attention to the chocolate, too. Quiz him a week later, and he will underreport what he ate.

## The Thyroid Gland

Many obese people believe that their obesity is due to an "underactive thyroid." They are usually wrong. Underactivity of the thyroid, or hypothyroidism, is not a cause of significant obesity.

The thyroid gland is located in the neck, in the position where a man knots his tie. The gland is shaped like a butterfly, thinnest in the middle and spreading out like wings on either side of the windpipe. You can easily put your fingers on it, but it is very hard to feel the gland unless it is enlarged or bumpy. An enlarged thyroid gland is called a goiter.

The thyroid gland produces thyroid hormone, which circulates in the blood and acts on most organs of the body to set the rate at which cells burn food to make heat. Patients with elevated thyroid function (hyperthyroidism) have low-grade fever, fast heartbeat, tremor, and weight loss. Patients with low thyroid function (hypothyroidism) have the opposite: low body temperature, slow heart rate, sluggishness, and sore muscles.

Hypothyroid patients do put on a little weight, but not as much as many people suppose. Even many physicians are confused about this. Hypothyroidism might account for 10 pounds of extra weight, at most, in a 240-pound hypothyroid patient. Most of that 10 pounds is extra body fluid, not fat.

Hypothyroidism occurs in only 2 percent of the general population. Obesity occurs in 35 percent. It should be obvious that hypothyroidism is not a significant cause of obesity.

*Hypothyroidism occurs in only 2 percent of the general population. Obesity occurs in 35 percent.*

Nevertheless, obese patients often beg their physician to perform blood tests to check for hypothyroidism, hoping the condition can be diagnosed so they can peel off the pounds by taking a simple hormone supplement. Life should be so kind! If hypothyroidism is diagnosed, patients must take a hormone supplement, but they must still deal with their obesity in the same way as obese patients with normal thyroid function.

A few decades ago, some doctors treated obesity by giving thyroid hormone to patients with normal thyroid function, intentionally inducing hyperthyroidism. The patients lost weight at the price of nervousness, tremor, and sweating. No ethical doctor today would give thyroid hormone to an obese patient with a normal thyroid. Hyperthyroidism is known to cause long-term harmful effects: it thins the heart and causes osteoporosis.

Thyroid function should be tested at an early stage of the phen-Prozac program, not because therapy for obesity can be bypassed, but because weight loss is slowed if the patient has unrecognized hypothyroidism.

## Cholesterol

Most people believe that obese people tend to have high cholesterol levels and thin people tend to have low cholesterol levels, but this is hardly true. The most important determinant of blood cholesterol level is your parents—the genetic factor. The second most important determinant is gender; women tend to have lower cholesterol levels than men. Diet is the third most important item on the list, and not a significant cause of high cholesterol level. Obesity is the least important factor on the list.

The reason is that there is a cholesterol "thermostat" in the liver. As a matter of fact, you can scarcely lower your cholesterol level by consuming less cholesterol because the liver responds to the "deficiency" by making more cholesterol! You can lower your blood cholesterol level by consuming less saturated fat—the starting material from which cholesterol is made—but this is hard to do.

Let's suppose the liver devotes 1 percent of dietary saturated fat to making cholesterol—that's approximately correct. If you reduce your intake of saturated fat by 50 percent—a nearly superhuman effort—the liver directs 2 percent of the saturated fat intake to cholesterol synthesis, instead of 1 percent, and the amount of cholesterol entering the bloodstream remains the same.

The National Institutes of Health (NIH) has recommended that we all get our total cholesterol count under 200. The borderline range is 200–240. Patients in this range are at some increased risk of heart disease and stroke, but they can reasonably get their cholesterol level below 200 with the small changes afforded by an improved diet. Patients with cholesterol levels over 240 are unlikely to get their cholesterol under 200 with any change in diet that an American is willing to make. Patients with two or more fasting cholesterol measurements in this range should be placed on cholesterol-lowering medication.

The NIH recommendations have stood the test of time. In 1997 we are more certain than ever that these guidelines are valid. It is a different story when we come to the official recommendations for a cholesterol-lowering diet.

In the early eighties, a group of physicians at the American Heart Association (AHA) debated and agreed on a set of dietary recommendations intended to reduce the national cholesterol level. The American Heart Association Diet was widely publicized.[1] Many AHA Diet cookbooks were published. Restaurants were inspected and certified as serving fare consistent with the AHA guidelines; conforming restaurants paid a fee and received a little red heart-shaped decal to display on their windows. The Walt Disney Company proudly declared that they had converted the restaurants in their theme parks to the AHA Diet.

All this effort was made, and no one checked to see if the diet really worked—until 1993, when the Medical College of Wisconsin published a study that showed that the Stage I AHA Diet made no significant difference on blood cholesterol levels. The stricter Stage II diet, intended for patients with established heart disease, made a more appreciable difference.

Obese patients with high cholesterol levels should not expect their cholesterol level to go down much due to the lower food intake and weight loss resulting from the phen-Prozac program. If the fasting cholesterol level is over 240, patients on the program should take a cholesterol-lowering medication in addition to phen-Prozac.

Don't be fooled by articles about "controversy" among doctors regarding whether high cholesterol should be treated. There is no controversy among true physicians on the subject. The association of high cholesterol with heart disease is a settled issue everywhere except in the pages of *Reader's Digest*.

## HDL Cholesterol

High-density lipoprotein (HDL) is the component of cholesterol that protects the heart from hardening of the arteries (atherosclerosis). It has been in the news a lot lately. In the bloodstream, cholesterol is transported on different particles.

Cholesterol molecules may wind up in various places, depending on which type of particle they adhere to. Low-density lipoprotein (LDL) particles originate in the liver and transport cholesterol to the muscles. Muscles do need some cholesterol; it has some legitimate uses in the body. The trouble is that some LDL gets stuck in artery walls, causing atherosclerosis. This phenomenon occurs naturally in only two species on earth: people and pigs.

HDL particles pick up cholesterol from the muscles, then transport them back to the liver to be excreted. The liver can synthesize cholesterol, but no organ in the body can break it down. Because cholesterol is not water-soluble, the only way to get rid of it is to dump it into the stool.

In addition to picking up cholesterol from the muscles, the HDL also picks up cholesterol from the arterial walls. Therefore, HDL reduces atherosclerosis. The higher the HDL level, the better.

*If your body is shaped like a pear, your HDL level tends to be high and your risk of heart attack low.*

The best indicator of heart attack risk is the ratio of the levels of total cholesterol to HDL. If the ratio is greater than 8, you're in great shape. If the ratio is less than 4, you are a time bomb. If you also smoke, you are a smoking time bomb.

The most important determinant of HDL levels is your parents (here we go again!). The second most important factor is your gender. Women tend to have higher HDL levels, because estrogen raises HDL levels. That's one major reason why women outlive men by eight years in the United States. (The other reasons are that women tend not to buy as many guns, drink as heavily, or drive as dangerously as men.)

*If your body is shaped like an apple, you are at greater risk because you are likely to have a low HDL level.*

The third important contributor to raising HDL levels is aerobic exercise. This is one reason I recommended exercise in Chapter 9, even though the usual amounts of exercise contribute little to weight loss. A little exercise contributes a lot to raising the HDL level. Several studies have demonstrated that thirty minutes of vigorous aerobic exercise three times a week produces two-thirds of the possible improvement in HDL level. Becoming a marathon runner adds only another one-third. So even a little exercise helps.

The fourth factor in raising HDL levels is losing excess body fat. One interesting study showed that the ratio of the diameter of the waist to the diameter of the hips was as good a predictor of heart attack risk as the blood cholesterol level. I suspect that it is not an independent predictor, however. Although obese patients do not necessarily have high cholesterol levels, they do tend to have low HDL levels. This is especially true if their extra body fat is stored around their middle. Fat stored around the hips is not very active metabolically, so it contributes little to lowering HDL.

These facts have resulted in the "apple and pear" analogy. If your body is shaped like a pear (widest at the hips), your HDL level tends to be high and your risk of heart attack low, provided other risk factors aren't present. If your body is shaped like an apple (widest at the waist), you are at greater risk because you are likely to have a low HDL level.

But nature is good to us. Remember, weight around the waist is easiest to lose. So the first pounds lost on phen-Prozac come from the area most important in reducing heart attack risk.

CHAPTER TWELVE

# Doctor to Doctor

*I will follow that system of regimen which, according to my ability and judgment, I consider for the benefit of my patients, and abstain from whatever is deleterious and mischievous.*

From the Hippocratic Oath, administered to physicians since 400 B.C.

Please share this chapter with your doctor to introduce him or her to the topic of medical weight-loss therapy. It contains information a physician needs to determine which prescription would work best for you.

## Overview

This book recommends a variant form of the popular "phen-fen diet," a combination of two, old, different, FDA-approved appetite suppressants: phentermine and fenfluramine. In the beginning phen-fen was the first truly effective, long-term medical treatment for obesity. The novel part of its premise was the idea of using two appetite suppressants together, as neither medicine worked well for very long, when used alone.

Relatively little about the treatment has been published in peer-reviewed journals; most physicians have heard about phen-fen only through the popular press and have, therefore, developed a negative reaction. Physicians are traditionally resistant to ideas in the popular press that sound "too good to be true."

This time, however, the idea really is good. There is no other truly effective long-term cure for obesity. Voluntary dieting and exercise programs don't work for long, as experience has probably told you!

The reason that there have been so few studies of phen-fen in medical journals is that both medicines in the combination are generics. No pharmaceutical company has been interested in funding phen-fen research, preferring to promote single agents that are 1) more profitable, and 2) easier to get approved by the FDA than a combination product. The original article on phen-fen was published by Dr. Michael Weintraub in *Clinical Pharmacology and Therapeutics* (1992; 51:581–585), a well-done, but small, double-blind, placebo-controlled trial with dramatic results.

Redux is a recently approved single agent, actually a better tolerated form of fenfluramine. You might think that giving Redux (fenfluramine) alone would not work as well as giving both phentermine and fenfluramine.

During 1996, approximately six million obese patients in the United States were started on phen-fen and three million on Redux. The patients on phen-fen refilled their prescriptions an average of three times.

While the large majority of patients on phen-fen and Redux will benefit, there is a hitch: fenfluramine, whether dispensed as Pondimin or Redux, can cause primary pulmonary hypertension (PPH) and mitral valve sclerosis. As of May 1997, the Centers for Disease Control is aware of one death in Massachusetts and a dozen other cases of fenfluramine-associated PPH. The Mayo Clinic has reported twenty-four cases of fenfluramine-associated mitral valve sclerosis. The issue has captured the attention of the press, and it may be difficult or unwise to continue prescribing fenfluramine.

This book describes a new combination treatment, phen-Prozac, which does not involve risk of PPH, and it works just as well for obesity as phen-fen. Only a very low dose of Prozac is required, and several other SSRI drugs can be substituted for Prozac, so the physician has much better control of potential side effects. I have written an article on my results with phen-Prozac for *Archives of Internal Medicine.*[1] That article and this book are currently the best sources you will find for information on phen-Prozac.

Medical therapy for obesity is a valid approach to take, now that it is known that the tendency to overeat is driven by abnormal brain chemistry. If you have considered phen-fen, but are worried about inducing PPH with fenfluramine, I suggest that phen-Prozac offers the soft spot between the rock and the hard place.

## Indications for Phen-Prozac

Postpubertal patients with a body mass index (BMI) in excess of 30 who have not been able to lose weight and keep weight off by the usual means of diet and exercise are the targeted candidates for this treatment. Patients may also be treated if their BMI is over 27 and they have obesity-related medical conditions that would be ameliorated by loss of weight.

The BMI may be calculated using the following formula:

$$\text{BMI} = \frac{\text{weight in pounds} \times 700}{\text{height in inches} \times \text{height in inches}}$$

A BMI between 19 and 25 is ideal. A BMI between 25 and 30 constitutes non-medical obesity. A BMI over 30 corresponds to morbid obesity and increased risks for obesity-related health problems.

## The Initial Dose

Phentermine generic 15 mg by mouth every morning with breakfast for one week *and* Prozac 10 mg (or 1/2 of 50-mg Zoloft) every day.

After one week, increase phentermine dose to 30 mg with breakfast.

Generic phentermine can be used because: 1) the brand-name product costs four times as much as the generic, and 2) the generic has a better time course of action than the brand-name products, which are time-released, leading to a lower blood level at lunch when an appetite suppressant action is needed and a higher blood level at bedtime, interfering with sleep. Generic phentermine with breakfast affords the ideal time course in most people.

It is extremely important to start with 15 mg of phentermine for the first week before increasing to 30 mg, even though most patients will require 30 mg for weight loss. Patients who start right away on 30 mg can be prone to nervousness and insomnia. I have found that when the phentermine is started slowly, these side effects are diminished or avoided altogether. The brain takes a little time to adapt to phentermine.

The lowest dose of Prozac (or Zoloft, or other SSRI, depending on the case) is usually sufficient for weight loss, but if the patient has any co-existing condition (such as depression, OCD, PMS) for which Prozac or Zoloft is used as treatment, higher doses of Prozac or Zoloft may be more beneficial.

Prozac and Zoloft have long half-lives; it takes a week or more to reach steady-state levels. Some side effects of Prozac and Zoloft appear immediately; others won't appear until a week or more after therapy has begun.

Phentermine and Prozac/Zoloft are not addictive. Phentermine is no longer classified as a Schedule III drug. Nevertheless, do not add a refill to the initial prescription, to ensure that the patient will return for follow-up.

## Absolute Contraindications for Phen-Prozac or Phen-Zoloft

---

bladder outlet obstruction due to enlarged prostate
congestive heart failure, grade II or worse
diabetes mellitus in poor control
epilepsy
family history of pulmonary hypertension
glaucoma
history of allergy or intolerance to the medications

history of drug abuse
history of vasospastic phenomena
hyperthyroidism, uncontrolled
litigious nature of the patient
residence in a state where phentermine use is prohibited
mania
myocardial infarction within the last six months
schizophrenia
severe hypertension
tachycardias (other than sinus tachycardia)

## Relative Contraindications for Phen-Prozac or Phen-Zoloft

chronic anxiety
enlarged prostate
gallstones
history of medical non-compliance
moderate hypertension
personal objection to use of drugs to treat obesity
sinus tachycardia

The reason for the warnings regarding the prostate is that phentermine, like any $\alpha$-agonist, can cause swelling of the prostate, precipitating bladder outlet obstruction in a patient with previously enlarged prostate. Gallstones can form or enlarge in the course of any successful weight-loss program; patients should be warned about this.

Phentermine does not raise blood pressure when used in the manner advocated in this book. Nor is phentermine addictive in moderate doses, but not every medical regulator knows that. Some of the contraindications in the previous list are more legal than medical, to protect the physician. As physicians gain experience with phen-Prozac and public acceptance increases, some of these restrictions can be dropped.

## Initial Lab Workup

A fasting blood glucose test should be done initially to detect undiagnosed diabetes. A postprandial urinalysis may suffice. If the patient is known to have diabetes mellitus, a glycohemoglobin A1C should be done to assess the degree of diabetic control. If the fasting blood sugar is over 180 mg% or the glycohemoglobin A1C is over 7.0%, a phen-Prozac program should be deferred until the patient's health is brought under better control with diet and other medication. In Type II diabetics, the addition of Glucophage to glyburide/glipizide is very effective, and may be preferable to raising the dose of glyburide/glipizide.

The patient may have a TSH (thyroid-stimulating hormone) test drawn initially to look for hypothyroidism, because hypothyroid patients have poor success with phen-Prozac therapy. Alternatively, the clinician may wait to see if the phen-Prozac program is a success, before obtaining the TSH test.

If there is any evidence of an obesity-producing metabolic disorder on exam or history,[2,3] the diagnosis should be sought before the patient is initiated on phen-Prozac.

Intraocular pressure measurement should be performed before inception of treatment, because uncontrolled glaucoma is a contraindication to phen-Prozac treatment.

## Concomitant Medications

Phentermine should not be taken together with a β-blocker because β-blockers block the anorectic effect of phentermine.[4] Phentermine should not be used with theophylline or oral α-agonists in asthma patients because of additive side effects. Inhaled α-agonists are acceptable.

Patients should be counseled not to drink coffee with caffeine when taking phentermine. The use of caffeine with phentermine increases the chance of stimulant side effects. Coffee does not have to contain caffeine to taste good anymore, now that coffee is decaffeinated with the Swiss (hot water) method. Decaffeinated colas are also available. The quantity of theophylline in tea is negligible compared to the level of caffeine in coffee, so the use of tea is fine.

Phentermine serves as a nasal decongestant. There is no need for a patient to take both a nasal decongestant and phentermine.

Phentermine is an adequate replacement for Ritalin in patients with ADD. Ritalin, on the other hand, is a poor appetite suppressant. Note: phentermine is not adequate therapy for narcolepsy.

Until more study is done, Prozac and other SSRIs should never be combined with another serotonergic agonist. The most common way in which this error is made is when Prozac is combined with fenfluramine in obese patients with depression, or when Sansert is given to obese patients with migraine. There is said to be a rare, but serious, "serotonin syndrome" in which patients taking too many serotonergic medicines are affected with extreme agitation, confusion, fever, and tachycardia.

When patients on more than 10 mg of Prozac are placed on erythromycin-like antibiotics, the Prozac dose should be reduced because both erythromycin and Prozac are metabolized by the cytochrome P-450 system in the liver. If the Prozac dose is not reduced during the course of erythromycin, the blood level of Prozac will increase, which may present a problem for some individuals. The usual caveat applies: if the patient is sick enough to need erythromycin, he or she is probably too sick to overeat anyway. Diet medications are not needed during an illness.

Phentermine should be discontinued two weeks before surgery involving general or regional anesthesia, because prolonged use of phentermine depletes peripheral catecholamines. If phentermine is not discontinued sufficiently before surgery, hypotension may ensue after induction of anesthesia.

## Safety During Pregnancy and Nursing

Prozac is the only SSRI for which there are enough data to show safety during pregnancy.[5] Other SSRIs are still a question mark. The effect of phentermine on pregnancy is unknown. Female patients on phen-Prozac should be advised to use contraception. If they miss a menstrual period while on phen-Prozac, a pregnancy test should be obtained. If the patient is found to be pregnant, phentermine should be discontinued. Prozac may be continued if needed for depression.

It is not known whether phentermine or the SSRIs other than Prozac are safe in nursing. The wisest course would be to delay phen-Prozac treatment until after the period of nursing.

## Diet and Exercise

Initial exercise advice should be tailored to the specific situation of the individual patient. Very obese patients should be encouraged to exercise in water or in low-impact activities, such as a treadmill, to protect the knees. Patients in better condition can do more vigorous exercises. Patients should exercise to the point where the heart rate is increased but they are not short of breath (aerobic exercise). Exercise should be stopped if chest pain develops, and the physician should be contacted immediately. Smokers and other patients with elevated cardiovascular risk should undergo a cardiology workup before starting an exercise program.

My diet advice for the patients is simple:

1. Don't eat when you are not hungry. Eat slowly and stop eating when you feel full.
2. Don't buy what you shouldn't eat.
3. Eat your largest meal in the middle of the day.
4. Fill your plate with low-calorie side dishes first. Only when you have eaten a full plate of these items should you venture to fill your plate with the main course.
5. Cut back on foods that come from land animals.
6. Eat foods that are spicier and more aromatic.
7. Don't eat in restaurants so often. When you do eat out, choose restaurants that serve smaller servings or share dishes with others.
8. If you are drinking too much alcohol, cut back or get help.

Patients should not take phen-Prozac on days when they are not eating due to an illness or a religious fast. Patients should discontinue phentermine two weeks before elective surgery, to avoid hypertension during anesthesia.

## Plan of Follow-Up

See the patient in the office seven to ten days after the initial visit to ensure that the patient has comfortably negotiated the transition from 15 mg to 30 mg of phentermine and that the patient is not experiencing agitation or confusion. These side effects are very uncommon. If they occur on inception of treatment, they are a result of the phentermine. If they occur a week or more later, they are probably a consequence of the Prozac/Zoloft. If the patient is agitated, both medications should be stopped. Agitation from Prozac/Zoloft will take several days to wear off because of the long half-life.

Thereafter, schedule follow-up visits with the patient every four to six weeks. Weigh the patient each time and ask about side effects. Expect them to lose about 1 to $1^1/_2$ pounds per week. There is no limit on how long phen-Prozac may be given. The goal should be a BMI of 25, if it can be achieved. Otherwise, a BMI of 27 can be accepted as a target of opportunity.

After starting the medication, one of four things may happen (refer to Figure 12.1):

1. The patient may lose no weight in spite of the medicines, diet, and exercise (Curve A).
2. The patient may lose weight very slowly (Curve B).
3. The patient may lose weight quickly at first, and slow down later (Curve C).
4. The patient may lose weight and keep on losing (Curve D).

**Possible Outcomes Using Phen-Prozac**

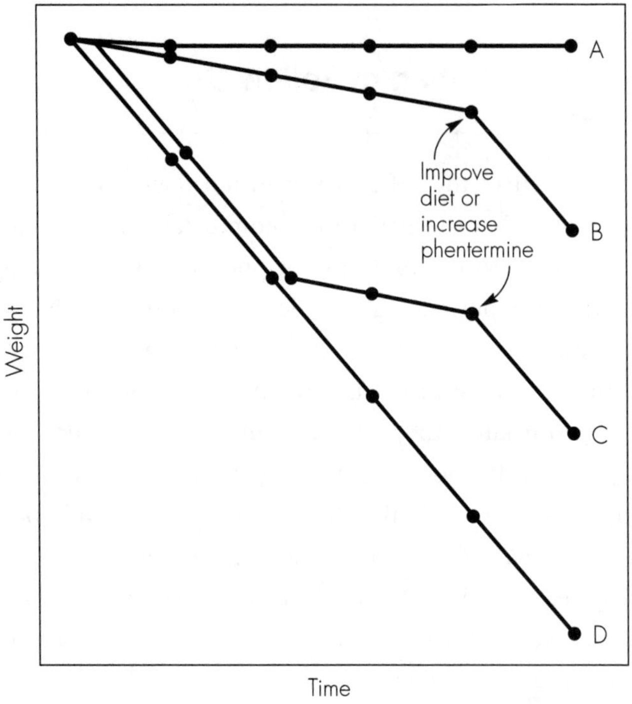


FIGURE 12.1

If the patient is on a plateau for three weeks or more, encourage the patient to pay more rigorous attention to diet and exercise. If this doesn't work, the next step is to increase the dose of phentermine by 15 mg, to a maximum of 60 mg per day. A dose of 45 mg may be taken all at once in the morning or divided between breakfast and lunch. A dose of 60 mg should always be split between breakfast and lunch.

Phentermine is available as a generic medication in two dosage strengths: 15 mg and 30 mg. The generic is much cheaper than the brand-name versions, and actually has a better time course of action. Brand-name versions are Ionamin and Fastin. Phentermine is also available as Adipex, 37.5 mg. Adipex is the hydrochloride salt of phentermine; 37.5 mg of Adipex is equivalent to 30 mg of phentermine base.

Do not change the phentermine prescription to Dexedrine to scale up the appetite suppressant effect. Dexedrine is a potent addictive medication closely watched by regulatory agencies.

If the patient is not losing weight at the desired rate, ask what time the patient is taking the medicine. If it is with breakfast in the wee hours of the morning because his or her job starts early, try moving the time to midmorning with a snack, or before lunch.

A small dose of Prozac/Zoloft suffices for maximum weight loss. Some dose of Prozac/Zoloft must be given with the phentermine if you want to achieve sustained weight loss. Don't give phentermine alone without good reason. Most patients develop tachyphylaxis on phentermine alone.

If the patient has co-existing depression, the Prozac dose may be administered at 20 mg (or Zoloft 50–100 mg) to control the depression. If the patient has severe OCD, the Prozac dose may be raised stepwise to 40–60 mg to control the OCD. If the patient has any serious psychiatric disorder, I do not advise prescribing appetite suppressant therapy without consulting a psychiatrist first, for both medical and legal reasons.

There are many possible side effects of phen-Prozac. Most will abate with time; patience is a virtue. The following list details the side effects of phen-Prozac seen in 535 patients, frequency with which the side effects were seen, and measures found to reduce or eliminate them:

| Side Effect | Effective Responses |
|---|---|
| *Frequent (more than 30 percent of patients)* | |
| dry mouth | drink more fluids<br>suck on lemon drops<br>chew gum |
| sweating | wear cooler clothing<br>Drysol for feet or axillae<br>spray body with anti-perspirant for total body sweating |
| *Moderately Frequent (10–30 percent of patients)* | |
| trouble falling asleep | take phentermine earlier in day<br>lower dose of phentermine<br>cut out caffeine |
| trouble staying asleep | lower dose of Prozac/Zoloft<br>substitute trazodone, 50 mg qhs |
| nervousnes | lower dose of phentermine<br>cut out caffeine |
| drowsiness | lower phentermine dose<br>take Prozac/Zoloft at night |
| decreased sex drive<br>orgasmic delay[6] | substitute Luvox 50 mg for Prozac/Zoloft |
| constipation | increase fiber and fluids<br>lower dose of phentermine |

| Side Effect | Effective Responses |
|---|---|
| *Rare (fewer than 10 percent of patients)* | |
| tachycardia | lower dose of phentermine<br>cut out caffeine |
| diarrhea | lower dose of Prozac/Zoloft<br>Kaopectate<br>apples, bananas |
| headache | lower dose of either phentermine or SSRI |
| partial amnesia (often a result of decreased sleep or decreased dreaming) | switch SSRI to trazodone at hs |

## Goal Weight

The patient should continue phen-Prozac until one of the following occurs:

- the desired goal weight or a body mass index of 25 is reached, whichever comes first
- a plateau is reached, beyond which further weight loss cannot be induced by improved diet or exercise or increasing the dose of phentermine
- intolerable side effects intervene
- the patient wants to stop

You need not worry that weight will decrease so precipitously that the patient will pass through the zone of normal weight and become too thin before the therapy is stopped. The patient's body weight approaches ideal asymptotically. The easiest pound to lose is always the first, and the hardest to lose is the last. The therapy will not reduce the weight of normal-weight individuals further.

## Maintenance Therapy

Once the patient achieves goal weight, phen-Prozac should be stopped for a trial period of four weeks. Advise the patient to continue a reasonable low-fat diet and exercise plan during the trial period. When the patient returns to the office after four weeks, if the weight has remained approximately the same, no further follow-up visits need to be scheduled. It should be emphasized that if the patient starts to gain weight in the future, the physician should be contacted.

If the patient gains weight during the trial period, maintenance drug therapy can be offered. My practice is to prescribe a supply of 15-mg phentermine and 10-mg Prozac capsules and tell the patient to take the medicines with the least frequency necessary to keep weight constant. Some patients take the medicines every other day; others take it every day for one or two weeks out of the month. They may increase the medication during holidays and vacations and decrease it during illnesses or religious fasts. Patients on maintenance therapy should be followed infrequently but regularly. Reminder cards should be sent for scheduled follow-ups.

## The Last Word

Having read this chapter, you will know as much about phen-Prozac therapy as about any other therapy given in the office. Other medical authorities in the future may develop even better ways to deliver combination appetite suppressant therapy, but if phen-Prozac is the only method you ever learn, I am confident it will serve as an adequate basis for therapy for 95 percent of obese patients for a long time to come.

# Appendix

**Natural neurotransmitters:**

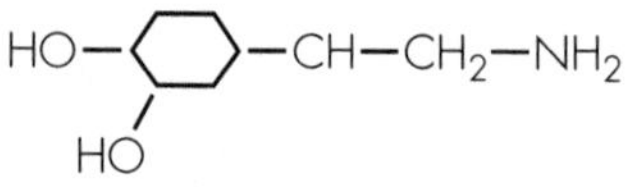

dopamine

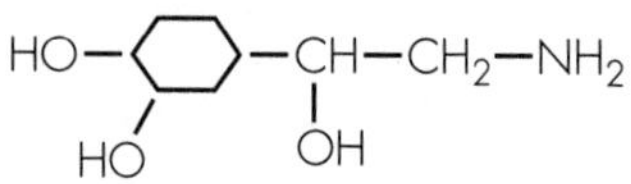

norepinephrine

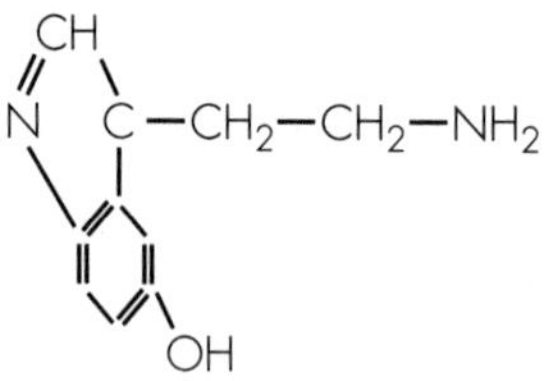

serotonin

**Drugs that resemble norepinephrine:**

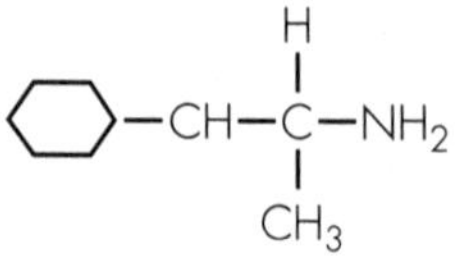

Dexedrine

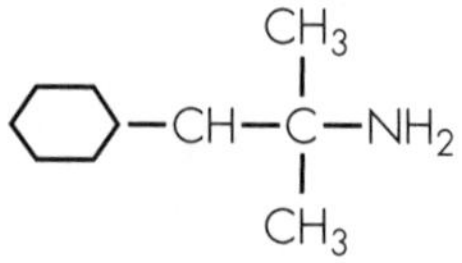

phentermine

## Drugs that resemble serotonin and work with phentermine to produce weight loss:

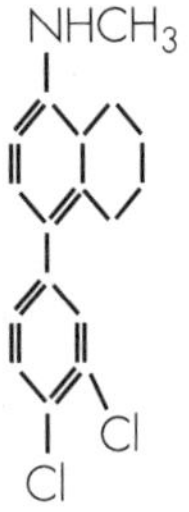

Zoloft

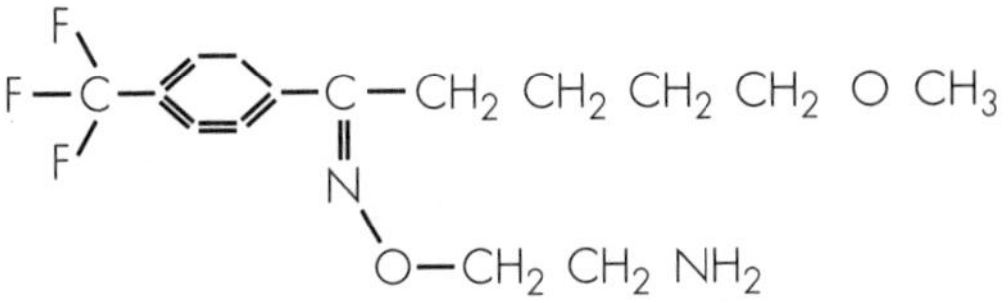

Luvox

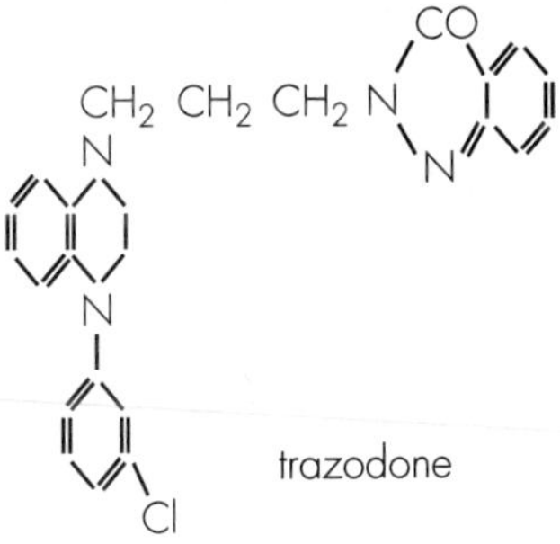

trazodone

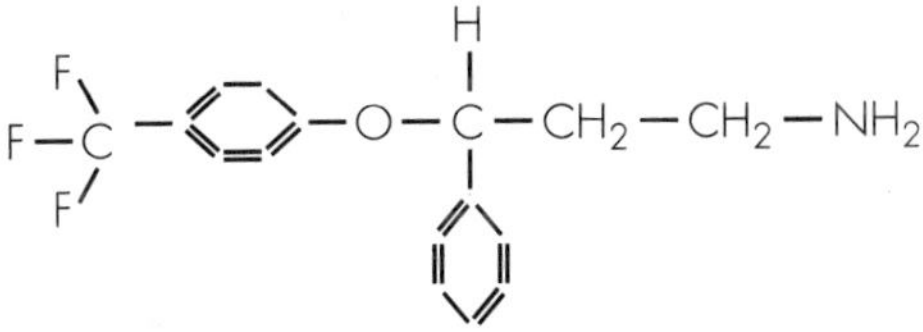

Prozac

## Drugs that can cause primary pulmonary hypertension (PPH):

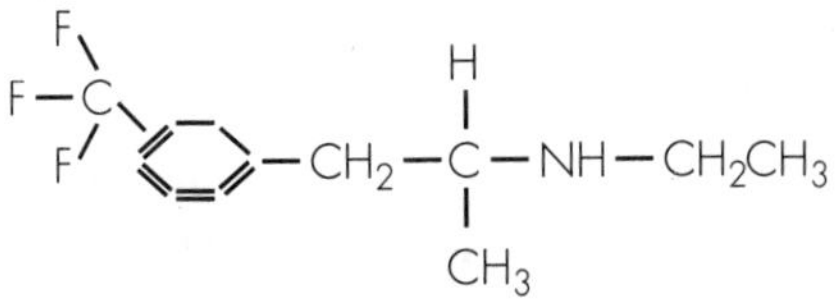

fenfluramine, Redux, Pondimin

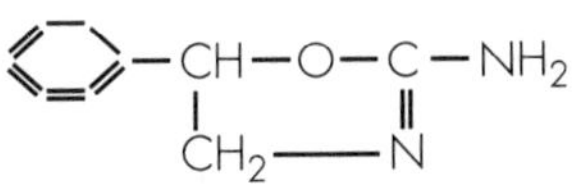

Aminorex

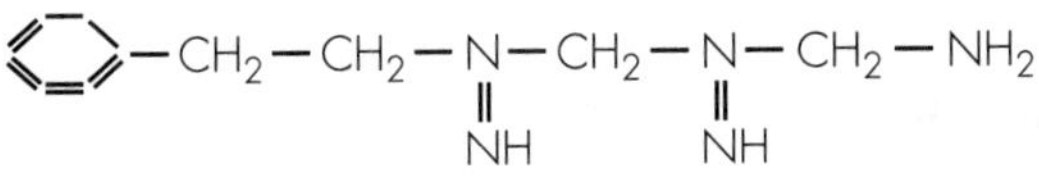

phenformin

# Notes


**Chapter One**

1. Abenhaim, L. et al., "Appetite-Suppressant Drugs and the Risk of Primary Pulmonary Hypertension." *New England Journal of Medicine* 335 (1996): 609–16.

2. Anchors, M., "Fluoxetine Is a Safer Alternative to Fenfluramine in the Medical Treatment of Obesity." *Archives of Internal Medicine* 157 (1997): 1270.

3. Abernathy, R.P. et al., "Is Adipose Tissue Oversold As a Health Risk?" *Journal of the American Dietetic Association* 94 (1994): 641–49.

4. Manson, J. et al., "Body Weight and Mortality Among Women." *New England Journal of Medicine* Sup. 1 (1995): 2 04.

5. Gortmacher, S.L. et al., "Social and Economic Consequences of Overweight in Adolescence and Young Adulthood." *New England Journal of Medicine* 329 (1994): 1008–12.

6. Health, Education, and Welfare Conference on Obesity, 1973. Heights are without shoes, weights without clothes.

7. Eck, L.H. et al., "Physicians' Diagnosis of Obesity . . ." and other articles in *Journal of Obesity-Related Metabolic Disorders* 18 (1994): 503–12, 704–8.

8. Kuczmarski, R. et al. "Increasing Prevalence of Overweight Among U.S. Adults, the National Health and Nutrition Examination Surveys, 1960–1991." *Journal of American Medical Association* 272 (1994): 205–12.

9. Centers for Disease Control, *Morbidity and Mortality Weekly Report,* cited in *Washington Post,* (March 7, 1997).

10. Levine, Sheldon, M.D., *The Redux Revolution.* (William Morrow and Company. New York: 1996).

**Chapter Two**

1. Blundell, J.E. et al., "Mechanisms of Appetite Control and Their Abnormalities on Obese Patients." *Hormonal Research* 39, Sup. 3 (1993): 72–76.

2. Leibowitz, S.F. et al., "Neurochemical/Neuroendocrine Systems in the Brain Controlling Macronutrient Intake and Metabolism." *Trends in Neuroscience* 15 (1992): 491–97.

3. Reaven, G.M., "Role of Insulin Resistance in Human Disease." *New England Journal of Medicine* 334 (1996): 324–25.

4. Lewis, D.E. et al., "Intense Exercise and Food Restriction Cause Similar Hypothalamic Neuropeptide Y Increases in Rats." *American Journal of Physiology* 264 (1993): 279–84.

5. Campfield, L.A. et al., "Recombinant Mouse Ob Protein: Evidence for a Peripheral Signal Linking Adiposity and Central Networks." *Science* 269 (1995): 546–549.

6. Montague, C.T. et al., "Congenital Leptin Deficiency Is Associated with Severe Early-Onset Obesity in Humans." *Nature* 387 (1997): 903–908.

7. Selikowitz, M., "Fenfluramine in Prader-Willi Syndrome: A Double-Blind, Placebo-Controlled Trial." *Archives of Diseases of Children* 65 (1990): 112–14.

8. I did not count these two women as "treatment failures." In Chapter 7, I state that I have had only seven treatment failures—phen-Prozac patients who did not lose weight—but that group did not include these lean women. I didn't think it fair to count them as failures.

**Chapter Three**

1. Lemonick, M. et al., "The New Miracle Drug?" *Time* (September 23, 1996): 61–67.

2. Wurtman, J.J. *The Serotonin Solution.* (Fawcett. Columbine, New York: 1996.).

3. Silverstone, T. et al. "A Comparative Evaluation of Dextrofenfluramine and dl-Fenfluramine on Hunger, Food Intake, Psychomotor Function and Side Effects in Normal Human Subjects," ed. A.E. Bender and L.J Brookes *Bodyweight Control: The Physiology, Clinical Treatment and Prevention of Obesity* (Churchhill Livingstone, 1987), 240–46.

4. Kuczmarski, R. et al., "Increasing Prevalence of Overweight among U.S. Adults: The National Health and Nutrition Examination Surveys, 1960–1991." *Journal of American Medical Association* 272 (1994): 205–12.

5. Manson, J. et al., "Body Weight and Mortality Among Women." *New England Journal of Medicine* 333 (1995): 677–85.

6. Weintraub, M., "Long-Term Weight Control: The National Heart, Lung, and Blood Institute Funded Multimodal Intervention Study." *Clinical Pharmacologic Therapy* 51(5) (1992): 581–646.

7. See note 6, Chapter 3.

8. Atkinson, R.L. et al., "Combination Drug Treatment of Obesity in a Practice Setting." *Obesity Research* Sup. 1 (1993): 2 04 .

9. Berlin, I. et al., "Is it Dexfenfluramine or Weight Loss That Reduces Blood Pressure and Noradrenergic Activity in Obese Patients?" *European Journal of Clinical Pharmacology* 44 (1993): 601–3.

10. "Obesity-Drug Duo Spurs Weight Loss and Maintenance." Medical Tribune of the *New York Times* 37, no. 7, April 4, 1996.

**Chapter Four**

1. Abenhaim, L. et al., "Appetite-Suppressant Drugs and the Risk of Primary Pulmonary Hypertension." *New England Journal of Medicine* 335 (1996): 609–16.

2. Rich, S. and B. H. Brundage, "Primary Pulmonary Hypertension." *Journal of the American Medical Association* 251 (1984): 2252–54.

3. Nall, K. C. et al., "Reversible Pulmonary Hypertension Associated with Anorexigen Use." *American Journal of Medicine* 91 (1991): 97–99.

4. Rich, S. et al., "Primary Pulmonary Hypertension: A National Prospective Study." *Annals of Internal Medicine* 107 (1987): 216–23.

5. See note 1, Chapter 4.

6. See note 2, Chapter 4.

7. Walcott, G. et al., "Primary Pulmonary Hypertension." *American Journal of Medicine* 49 (1970): 70–79.

8. McDonnell, P. J., et al., "Primary Pulmonary Hypertension and Cirrhosis: Are They Related?" *American Review of Respiratory Diseases* 127 (1983): 437–41.

9. See note 1, Chapter 4.

10. Garcia-Dorado, D. et al., "An Epidemic of Pulmonary Hypertension after Toxic Rapeseed Oil Ingestion in Spain." *Journal of the American College of Cardiology* 5 (1983): 1216–22.

11. Follath, F. et al., "Drug-Induced Pulmonary Hypertension?" *British Medical Journal* 1 (1971): 265–66.

12. Kay, J. M. et al., "Aminorex and the Pulmonary Circulation." *Thorax* 26 (1971): 262–70.

13. Fahlen, M. et al., "Phenformin and Pulmonary Hypertension." *British Heart Journal* 35 (1973): 824–28.

14. Herve, P. et al., "Increased Plasma Serotonin in Primary Pulmonary Hypertension." *American Journal of Medicine* 99 (1995): 249–54.

15. Weir, E.K. et al., "Anorexic Agents Aminorex, Fenfluramine, and Dexfenfluramine Inhibit Potassium Current in Rat Pulmonary Vascular Smooth Muscle and Cause Pulmonary Vasoconstriction." *Circulation* 94 (1996): 2216–20.

16. Douglas, J. G. et al., "Pulmonary Hypertension and Fenfluramine." *British Medical Journal* 283 (1981): 881–83.

17. Atanassott, P. G. et al., "Pulmonary Hypertension and Dexfenfluramine." *Lancet* 339 (1992): 436.

18. Brenot, F. et al., "Primary Pulmonary Hypertension and Fenfluramine Use." *British Heart Journal* 70 (1993): 537–41.

19. Lemonick, M. et al., "The New Miracle Drug?" *Time* (September 23, 1996).

**Chapter Five**

1. Medical Economics Data Production Company, *Physicians' Desk Reference,* 50th ed. Montvale, NJ: 1996.

2. Nash, Madeleine, "ADDICTED. Why do people get hooked? Mounting evidence points to a powerful brain chemical called dopamine." *Time* (May 5, 1997): 68–76.

3. Neergaard, Lauran, "FDA Approves Antidepressant as Anti-Smoking Drug." *Washington Post* (May 20, 1997): 11 (*Health*).

4. Bray, G. A., "A Case for Drug Treatment of Obesity." *Hospital Practice* 29 (1994): 53, 57–8. Dr. Bray is also quoted in *Journal of American Medical Association* 276 (1996): 1125–26.

5. Rothman, R. B., "Phentermine Pretreatment Antagonizes the Cocaine-Induced Rise in Mesolimbic Dopamine." *NeuroReport* 7(18) (1996): 25–26.

6. Rothman, R. B., Ayestas, M., Baumann, M. H. "Phentermine Pretreatment Antagonizes the Cocaine-Induced Rise in Mesolimbic Dopamine." *Neuroreport* 7:2–3.

7. Rothman, R. B., T. Gendron, and P. Hitzig, "Combined Use of Fenfluramine and Phentermine in the Treatment of Cocaine Addiction: A

Pilot Case Series." *Journal of Substance Abuse Treatment* (Letter) 11(3) (1994): 273–75.

8. Rothman, R. B., "Smoking Cessation in a Patient Being Treated with Fenfluramine Plus Phentermine for Simple Obesity." *Journal of Clinical Psychiatry* 57(2) (1996): 92–93.

9. Bray, G., "Barriers to the Treatment of Obesity." *Annals of Internal Medicine* (1991).

10. Anchors, M., "Fluoxetine Is a Safer Alternative to Fenfluramine in the Medical Treatment of Obesity." *Archives of Internal Medicine* 157 (1997): 1270.

**Chapter Six**

1. Teicher, M. H. et al., "Emergence of Intense Suicidal Preoccupation during Fluoxetine Treatment." *American Journal of Psychiatry* 147 (1990): 207–10.

2. Tolefson, G. D. et al., "Evaluation of Suicidality during Pharmacologic Treatment of Mood and Nonmood Disorders [Review]." *Annals of Clinical Psychiatry* 5 (1993): 209–24.

3. Fava, M. and J. F. Rosenbaum, "Suicidality and Fluoxetine: Is There a Relationship?" *Journal of Clinical Psychiatry* 52 (1991): 108–11.

4. Behar, R., "The Thriving Cult of Greed and Power." *Time* (May 6, 1991): 35.

5. Burton, T. M., "Anti-Depression Drug of Eli Lilly Loses Sales After Attack by Sect." *Wall Street Journal* (April 19, 1991).

6. Burton, T. M., "Panel Finds No Credible Evidence to Tie Prozac to Suicides and Violent Behavior." *Wall Street Journal* (September 23, 1991).

7. Burton, T. M., "Scientólogists Fail to Persuade FDA on Prozac." *Wall Street Journal* (August 2, 1991).

8. Cornwell, J. *The Power to Harm* (Viking Press. New York: 1996).

9. "Part 67: Medical Standards and Certification." *Federal Aviation Regulations*, (July 9, 1996).

10. Rothman, R. B., "Treatment of a Four-Year-Old Boy with ADHD with Phentermine." *Journal of Clinical Psychiatry* 57(7) (1996): 308–9.

11. Rothman, R. B., T. Gendron, and P. Hitzig, "Combined Use of Fenfluramine and Phentermine in the Treatment of Cocaine Addiction: A Pilot Case Series." *Journal of Substance Abuse Treatment* (Letter) 11(3) (1994): 273–75.

12. Rothman, R. B., "Smoking Cessation in a Patient Being Treated with Fenfluramine Plus Phentermine for Simple Obesity." *Journal of Clinical Psychiatry* 57(2) (1996): 92–93.

**Chapter Seven**

1. Personal communication from Dr. Richard Rothman.

2. Heber, David, L.J. Aronne, R. Blank, J. Foreyt, and D. Schumaker, "New Advances in the Treatment of Obesity." (videotape), American Medical Communications, Houston, Texas, (1997).

**Chapter Eight**

1. White, A. et al., *Principles of Biochemistry* (McGraw-Hill. New York: 1978).

2. Jeffery, R.W. et al., "A Randomized Trial of Counseling for Fat Restriction versus Calorie Restriction in the Treatment of Obesity." *International Journal of Obesity and Related Metabolic Disorders* 19 (1995): 132–37.

3. Lyon, X. H. et al., "Compliance to Dietary Advice Directed Towards Increasing the Carbohydrate-to-Fat Ratio of the Everyday Diet." *International Journal of Obesity and Related Metabolic Disorders* 19 (1995): 260–69.

4. Key, T. J. A. et al., "Dietary Habits and Mortality in 11,000 Vegetarians and Health-Conscious People: Results of a 17-Year Follow-Up." *British Medical Journal* 313 (1996): 775–79.

5. Data from the *American Almanac* (Hoover. Austin, Texas: 1996) citing the statistical abstract of the United States, 1994. Americans also drank 2.5 gallons of wine per person and 1.8 gallons of hard liquor.

6. Bread is not the "staff of life" in southern China. There have been so many people living on the land for so long that they have chopped down most of the trees. As a result, the Chinese don't have enough fuel to fire ovens. Ovens are inefficient; all the heat left in the bricks of the oven after baking is wasted energy. The Chinese use woks to make the best use of the remaining fuel. As a result of this choice of equipment, the southern Chinese can't bake bread; they use rice as a starch instead. In the northern part of China, in the Amur River Valley where forests still abound, the citizens do bake bread.

7. Pritikin, Nathan. *The Pritikin Program for Diet and Exercise* (Grosset and Dunlap. New York: 1979).

8. Atkins, Robert C., *Dr. Atkins' New Diet Revolution* (M. Evans & Company. New York: 1996).

9. Eades, Michael and Mary Dan, *Protein Power* (Bantam Books. New York: 1996).

10. Nutridata Software Company, 1988.

11. Some of the decrease in kidney function in Western countries could be due to the greater frequency of atherosclerosis—hardening of the arteries—causing obstruction of the renal arteries. Atheroscelorosis is more common in societies that consume a high-fat diet. Nevertheless, the influence of atherosclerosis should be more than offset by the frequency of tuberculosis and parasitic diseases affecting the kidneys in agrarian societies. The decline in kidney function in Western societies, as compared to agrarian societies, is still an enigma. It may be due to excess protein ingestion.

**Chapter Nine**

1. To be precise, the "equation" should be written:

$$\frac{\text{calories in} - \text{calories out}}{\text{3,600 calories/pound}} = \text{change in body fat}$$

2. A calorie is defined as the amount of heat required to raise the temperature of 1 gram of pure water 1 degree Celsius. It's a handy unit of measurement for physicists, but if dietitians used the calorie as their basic unit, they would have to deal with very large numbers—lots of zeros—so they use the Calorie (with a capital "C") instead. One of the dietitian's Calories (uppercase "C") equals 1,000 of the physicist's calories (lowercase "c"). In this book, we have used calories (lowercase "c") meaning dietitian's Calories, to conform to the current practice of other nutritionist authors. We could have used the correct scientific term "kilocalories" instead of "Calories," but then the United States could use the metric system like the rest of the world does, and it doesn't.

3. Older, less fit people take longer to shed a pound by jogging. Women take longer, because they have smaller leg muscles. How many forty-year-old men or women can run as fast as our young man in the example—seven miles per hour?

4. Leibowitz, S. F. et al., "Neurochemical/Neuroendocrine Systems in the Brain Controlling Macronutrient Intake and Metabolism." *Trends in Neuroscience* 15 (1992): 491–97.

5. Wartik, N., "Good News About Your Sex Life." *Glamour* (May 1997): 225.

**Chapter Ten**

1. *Diabetes mellitus* is not the only kind of diabetes. There is also *diabetes insipidus,* an unrelated endocrine disorder. Diabetes means "running

through" in Greek, and both of these diseases involve copious urination. Only patients with diabetes mellitus have sugar in the urine. Physicians in ancient Greece differentiated the two diseases by tasting the patient's urine. If it tasted sweet, they knew the patient would die slowly and could be helped by a spartan diet. (Did Athenian doctors call it a spartan diet? I wonder . . .) If the urine did not taste sweet, they knew that the patient would die quickly and nothing could be done to help. It was tough to be a physician in those days! I guess it was tough to be a patient too.

2. Felber, J. P. et al., "Metabolic Origin of Insulin Resistance in Obesity with and Without Type II (Non-Insulin Dependent) Diabetes Mellitus." *Diabetologia* 36 (1993): 1221–29.

**Chapter Eleven**

1. AHA Nutrition Committee, "American Heart Association Guidelines for Weight Management Program for Healthy Adults." *Heart Diseases and Stroke* 3 (1994): 221–28.

**Chapter Twelve**

1. Anchors, M., "Fluoxetine Is a Safer Alternative to Fenfluramine in the Medical Treatment of Obesity." *Archives of Internal Medicine* 157 (1997): 1270.

2. Examples of obesity-producing endocrine disorders are Cushing's disease and the Stein-Leventhal Syndrome (polycystic ovary disease).

3. One of my patients who had hyperprolactinemia was resistant to phen-Prozac, and I suspect this was due to the insulin-like properties of prolactin. The prolactin level need not be drawn at the inception of phen-Prozac treatment in patients without galactorrhea, but the test should be considered for female patients on phen-Prozac whose weight loss is unusually slow.

4. Dr. Richard Rothman disagrees with me on this. He uses low doses of propanolol to reduce the stimulant side effects of phentermine. But my experience has been that β-blockers block the appetite suppressants.

5. Pastuszak, A. et al., "Pregnancy Outcome Following First-Trimester Exposure to Fluoxetine (Prozac)." *Journal of the American Medical Association* 269 (1993): 2246–48.

6. Orgasmic delay may actually be advantageous in men. I have given Prozac to young men solely for premature ejaculation, with a 40 percent rate of success.

# Index